100 CASES
in General Practice

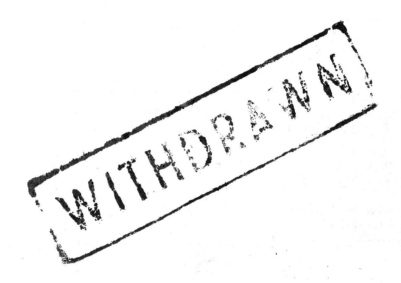

100 CASES
in General Practice

Anne Stephenson MBChB MRCGP PhD(Medicine) FHEA
Senior Lecturer in General Practice and Director of Community Education, King's
College London School of Medicine at Guy's, King's College and St Thomas' Hospitals,
London, UK

Martin Mueller MD MHPE MRCGP DCH DRCOG DIMC DFFP FHEA
Senior General Practice Tutor, King's College London School of Medicine at Guy's,
King's College and St Thomas' Hospitals, London; Visiting Senior Lecturer, Centre
for Medical Education, Barts and The London School of Medicine and Dentistry,
London, UK

John Grabinar BMBCh MRCGP MA(Oxon) DObstRCOG DCH
Lewisham Primary Care Trust, Lewisham, UK

100 Cases Series Editor:
P John Rees MD FRCP
Dean of Medical Undergraduate Education, King's College London School of Medicine
at Guy's, King's College and St Thomas' Hospitals, London, UK

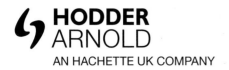

**HODDER
ARNOLD**

AN HACHETTE UK COMPANY

First published in Great Britain in 2009 by
Hodder Arnold, an imprint of Hodder Education, an Hachette UK Company,
338 Euston Road, London NW1 3BH

http://www.hoddereducation.com

British Library Cataloguing in Publication Data
A catalogue record for this book is available from the British Library

Library of Congress Cataloging-in-Publication Data
A catalog record for this book is available from the Library of Congress

ISBN   978 0 340 96833 8

1 2 3 4 5 6 7 8 9 10

Commissioning Editor: Sara Purdy
Project Editor: Eva Senior
Production Controller: Karen Dyer
Cover Designer: Amina Dudhia

Typeset in 10/12 RotiSerif by Macmillan Publishing Solutions. (www.macmillansolutions.com)
Printed and bound in India

What do you think about this book? Or any other Hodder Arnold title?
Please visit our website: www.hoddereducation.com

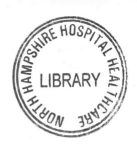

CONTENTS

PREFACE

We have chosen the following 100 cases in the hope that they are representative of the breadth and depth of general practice. People bring all kinds of matters to the general practitioner: those that pertain to health, illness and disease, and the physical, psychological, social and spiritual. As general practitioners we never know who will next come through our doors, and what they will bring.

When diagnosis is called for, our style is normally hypothetico-deductive and our questions sometimes ask you to decide on the differential diagnosis on the basis of the history we give you, and then to decide what line of further history-taking, focused examination, investigations and management you might take. Other scenarios are more classically inductive, presenting all the information first and then asking you to decide on the differential diagnosis and management; several are purely about management, communication or ethical considerations. We highlight the importance in our work of effective communication, continuity of care, team work and the necessity of placing patients' health issues in the context of their community and their life circumstances and experiences.

We have ordered these scenarios on the basis of the presenting symptom or topic: however, be aware that the presentation may have very little to do with what actually transpires. General practice consultations have a habit of not being what they first seem.

In general practice, listening is the key and the cases that are related in the following pages are from our experience as general practitioners: each scenario is an aggregate of many patients and many situations, and none is attributable.

'When I started in practice, the thing that gave me joy was the solving of clinical puzzles, the making of good diagnoses, thus impressing my colleagues. As time went on I found myself preoccupied more and more with the patients I had come to know. It was their joys and sorrows, their suffering and healing that moved me. Of course, clinical diagnosis and management did not cease to be crucial: simply that a patient's illness or disability became interwoven with a life story. I came to see medicine as more complex, more context-dependent, more poignant, more a reflection of the human condition'.

McWhinney, IR. Being a general practitioner: what it means.
Eur J Gen Pract 2006; 6: 135–9.

We hope that you will enjoy this book and that it will help to take you some way along this journey in understanding what general practice is about and how general practitioners approach the many and varied bio-psycho-social, cultural, and ethical issues encountered in everyday practice.

Anne Stephenson
Martin Mueller
John Grabinar
July 2008

ACKNOWLEDGEMENTS

The authors would like to thank Dr Richard Phillips for his expert assistance in deciding on the key points that we wished to get across in this volume. We are grateful to Jutta Warbruck for the illustrations of tongue conditions in Cases 16 and 67. We also thank Professor John Rees for his editing and Sara Purdy, Jane Tod and Eva Senior from Hodder Arnold for their encouragement.

ABBREVIATIONS

ACE	angiotensin-converting enzyme
AIDS	acquired immune deficiency syndrome
BCG	Bacille Calmette–Guérin (vaccine)
BMI	body mass index
BNP	B-type natriuretic peptide
BP	blood pressure
CCP	cyclic citrullinated peptides
CHD	coronary heart disease
CK	creatine kinase
COCP	combined oral contraceptive pill
COPD	chronic obstructive pulmonary disease
CRP	C-reactive protein
CT	computed tomography
CVA	cerebrovascular accident
CVD	cardiovascular disease
DAFNE	Dose Adjustment for Normal Eating programme
DMARD	disease-modifying anti-rheumatic drug
DTP	diphtheria/tetanus/pertussis (vaccine)
DVT	deep vein thrombosis
ECG	electrocardiogram
eGFR	estimated glomerular filtration rate
EPDS	Edinburgh Postnatal Depression Scale
ESR	erythrocyte sedimentation rate
FBC	full blood count
FEV_1	forced expiratory volume in 1 second
FSH	follicle-stimulating hormone
GFR	glomerular filtration rate
GP	general practitioner
Hb	haemoglobin
HDL	high-density lipoprotein
Hep B	hepatitis B (vaccine)
Hib	*Haemophilus influenzae* type b (vaccine)
HIV	*Human immunodeficiency virus*
HMG-CoA	3-hydroxy-3-methylglutaryl coenzyme A
1PV	poliomyelitis (vaccine)
JVP	jugular venous pressure
LH	luteinizing hormone
MCH	mean corpuscular haemoglobin
MenC	meningitis C (vaccine)
MMR	measles, mumps, rubella (vaccine)
MRI	magnetic resonance imaging
MSU	mid-stream urine

NHS	National Health Service
NICE	National Institute for Health and Clinical Excellence
NSAID	non-steroidal anti-inflammatory drug
PCOS	polycystic ovary syndrome
PCV	pneumococcal (vaccine)
PEG	percutaneous endoscopic gastrostomy
PET	positron-emission tomography
PHQ	Patient Health Questionnaire
PMR	polymyalgia rheumatica
PND	postnatal depression
POM	prescription-only medicine
POP	progesterone-only pill (mini-pill)
PSA	prostate-specific antigen
PTSD	post-traumatic stress disorder
QOF	Quality and Outcomes Framework
SCBU	Special Care Baby Unit
SLE	systemic lupus erythematosus
SSRI	selective serotonin reuptake inhibitor
TIA	transient ischaemic attack
TSH	thyroid-stimulating hormone
UTI	urinary tract infection

CASE 1: ABDOMINAL DISCOMFORT

History

The GP is consulted by a 58-year-old woman who presents with abdominal discomfort. Her symptoms are vague. The GP encourages her to explain. Over the past few months she has noticed an increasingly achy area in her left lower abdomen. Her abdomen also feels bloated. She has been passing urine more frequently and has been a bit constipated (unusual for her). She went through her menopause at 51 years of age but over the last week or two there has been a little vaginal spotting. Other than that she feels well and continues to work as a primary school teacher. She has been a healthy person and has not had any serious illnesses, has not smoked for many years and is a light alcohol drinker. Her smears have always been normal, the last one a year previously, and mammograms have also been normal. She lives with her husband and has one grown up daughter. She is an only child, her mother is still alive and well and her father died from lung cancer at 75 years of age.

The GP is worried that the symptoms that she describes could be something serious such as a tumour and asks her what she thinks could be going on. The GP knows that, if, as a result of the examination, they find a mass, then exploring the patient's concerns at this point of the consultation might make the breaking of possible bad news a little easier. The woman finds it difficult to express her worries. With some space and gentle encouragement she bursts into tears and tells the GP that she is worried that she has cancer and has been too afraid to come to the surgery to find out. The GP asks the patient whether she would like a family member, friend or chaperone to be present. The woman tells her that she would rather be there on her own and, if there is anything wrong, then she will deal with that later.

Examination

On abdominal examination the GP thinks she can feel a small, hard mass arising out of the pelvis and on vaginal examination there is a fixed left iliac fossa mass of about 6 cm in diameter. The most likely diagnosis is ovarian cancer.

Questions
- How might the GP break the bad news to the patient?
- What does the GP do now?

ANSWER

The woman can see that the GP is concerned. It is the middle of a busy morning but this is something that cannot be rushed. The other patients will have to wait and the GP asks the woman to get dressed and sit back down at the desk. The woman says to the GP 'It is cancer isn't it?' and the GP explains what she had found on the examination and that this is a possibility. The woman is quiet and very frightened and asks what should be done next and the GP tells her that it would be best if she was referred urgently under the 2-week rule to the local cancer services. The GP explains that it might not be cancer but that it would be best if proper investigations were carried out as soon as possible by a specialist unit. They talk about what the woman plans to do in the meantime. She is very concerned about telling her husband and daughter. She decides to go home and tell her husband who will be home at lunchtime and then, together, work out how to tell her daughter. She knows that her daughter will want to know straight away and would be very upset if she were not to hear until after the investigations. The GP arranges to see the couple again the next day at the end of the morning surgery.

Investigations did indeed show that she had ovarian cancer, Stage 3, and she went through surgery, chemotherapy and is in a period of remission.

Ovarian cancer is the fourth most common cancer among woman in the UK and there about 7000 new diagnoses each year. There are not usually symptoms in the early stages and unfortunately it is often detected late. Treatment is not usually curative. The aetiology is unknown: it is more common in nulliparous woman, less common in those women who have used the oral contraceptive pill, and rare in women under 30 years of age. In 5–10 per cent of women who have the disease there appears to be a major genetic component.

 KEY POINTS

- When symptoms or your intuition lead you to think that there may be something seriously wrong with your patient, prepare for possible bad news early in the consultation.
- Be as honest as you can: patients can tell when you are hiding something from them.
- Let patients lead the consultation: this makes it easier to explain what you suspect or know in a way that is best for them.
- Do not surrender patients totally to secondary services. It is important that you remain a support for them and their family.

CASE 2: ABDOMINAL PAIN

History

It is 7 p.m. on a Friday night in January. Evening surgery has finished and you are about to transfer the telephone to the weekend on-call service when a call comes in from the mother of three children, aged 3, 5 and 8 years. They have all had tummy-ache, diarrhoea and vomiting in the last 24 hours. They are normally healthy children, with only minor illnesses in the past. They have not been abroad recently and their mother and father are both well. The mother has already sensibly stopped them eating and has given them just water to drink, plus a dose of paracetamol to help the pain. You know there has been a minor outbreak of winter vomiting disease (*Norwalk virus*) locally. She is sorry to trouble you, and is merely seeking advice on how best to manage them.

Questions

- Do you need to visit the family?
- What further questions would help to answer this question?
- What advice should you offer to the mother?

ANSWER

The decision to make a home visit is the doctor's responsibility. It is perfectly reasonable, after taking an adequate history, to offer her simple advice (see below), and to ask her to contact the on-call service if any of the children do not improve as expected – perfectly reasonable, but not necessarily comfortable. You may well find yourself worrying about the case over the weekend, probably needlessly. Although homes are not ideal places for clinical examination, and home visits are time-consuming, they remain an essential part of the GP's duties. The decision to visit remains with the doctor, but we should consider the logistics from the patient's point of view. Imposing a car journey to an out-of-hours centre on this mother, with three vomiting children, would be contrary to their, and her, best interests, and would not foster that good patient–doctor relationship that we spend all our working lives trying to cultivate. We should learn to recognize our own very human feelings of irritation in this situation, and deal with the problem rationally.

You may ask some 'closed' questions to elucidate the problem. Is the abdominal pain constant, and does it prevent any of the children from getting up and running around? Are there any associated features, such as a rash, or fever?

Since all three are described as confined to bed you do visit, to find all three children in the parental bed, in various stages of misery. A forehead skin thermometer shows a low-grade fever in all of them. A gentle hand pressing on the abdomen reveals two who giggle, and one (the eldest) who moans. You ask them to try sitting up with their arms folded. You start with the eldest (as the others will copy the action) who cannot do this, while his younger brother and sister manage it easily.

You decide to admit the eldest to hospital, as a potential case of appendicitis. The other two can be managed with simple fluid replacement. A prescription for flavoured glucose–electrolyte powder, dissolved in 200 mL water and offered after every loose stool, is helpful. As they recover, they can supplement with starchy foods and even moderate amounts of 'crisps and cola' (salt and glucose).

A week later, you see all three in the surgery for follow-up. They have obviously recovered, and are 'bouncing' around the room. The eldest proudly shows his right iliac fossa scar, with subcuticular stitch awaiting removal by the practice nurse. Evidently, the hospital agreed with your diagnosis. The transient irritation of that Friday-night call is erased by the satisfaction of a job well done.

This problem highlights the dangers of assuming a diagnosis based on history and local epidemiology. It is safer to say 'there's a lot of it about' after you have examined the patient, rather than before.

 KEY POINTS

- Home visits remain an essential part of the general practitioner's duties.
- Do not assume a diagnosis based purely on history and local epidemiology.

CASE 3: ABDOMINAL PAIN

History
You are visited by a 22-year-old ceramics student at the local art college, who has been a patient of your practice since birth. He is a sensitive and studious young man, who lives with his parents and younger sister. His mother is an anxious intellectual, his father teaches at another college, and you have been concerned for some time that his 18-year-old sister might be anorexic. He has been experiencing sharp abdominal pains, poorly localized to the mid-zone, for some months, with occasional diarrhoea but no vomiting. He has tried antacids and paracetamol without success, and asks whether he should try a wheat- and dairy-free diet. He returned from a trip to Tanzania earlier this year.

Examination
He is a thin, almost asthenic, young man with no specific abnormalities in his abdomen.

INVESTIGATIONS
His urine shows no blood, sugar or protein.

You prescribe mebeverine as an antispasmodic, and see him in a week's time.

Questions
- What are the likely causes of his symptoms?
- What investigations would you suggest?
- How would you manage this case further?

ANSWER

> **!**
>
> Common things occur commonly. Viral gastroenteritis is still possible, although the recurrent symptoms make this less likely. Don't forget appendicitis. Irritable bowel syndrome is very common, and could be considered likely in view of his family and personal history of anxiety, but can only be posited after excluding other serious or treatable conditions. All returning travellers should be suspected of malaria or a bowel infection. His exposure to ceramic glazes might hint at lead colic: does he have a blue line on his gum? Renal or biliary colic, owing to calculi or infection, are possible. Coeliac disease is also a possibility and is often missed as it can present with any number of non-specific symptoms, most people with this disease are of normal weight or even overweight on presentation and it can be easily confused with irritable bowel syndrome.

A blood count, liver and renal function tests, serological tests for coeliac disease and an ultrasound scan of his abdomen would be helpful as would some stool samples looking for bacteria, ova, cysts and parasites. You may think of Crohn's disease or colitis, and suggest a colonoscopy, or barium radiography. In this case all tests were normal apart from raised endomysial antibodies pointing to coeliac disease and he was referred to a gastroenterologist for jejunal biopsy. He has greatly improved on a gluten-free diet, pre-scribable on the NHS and he now gets lifelong free prescriptions. Don't forget to call in his sister; your suspicion of anorexia may need to be revised: and what about his mother and father?

KEY POINTS

- Non-specific symptoms such as abdominal pain need an organized approach.
- Consider whether the traditional rectal examination is indicated here. Many patients find it intrusive and undignified, and it may not add to your clinical knowledge.
- Coeliac disease is considerably underdiagnosed in general practice so test for it with any patient with anaemia, tiredness or chronic abdominal symptoms.

CASE 4: ABDOMINAL PAIN

History

The GP is visited by a 30-year-old woman whom she knows well. The woman has a 2-day history of lower abdominal pain. The pain is low down in the right side of her abdomen and is constant and sharp, worse when she passes a bowel motion or sits down. Her periods normally come every 21–35 days and she has not had one this time for 40 days, although she has had some spotting for the past few days. She feels a little nauseated and her breasts are tender as if her period is about to arrive. She has been going to the toilet a little more frequently but it does not hurt when she passes urine and her urine does not appear cloudy or smell different from usual. Over the past day or two she has been feeling a little faint at times. She does not have a vaginal discharge and has not felt feverish. She has a long history of adenomyosis and pelvic inflammatory disease that has required many general practice and hospital visits and investigations. Recently, she has been much improved, her periods have been more regular and less heavy and her chronic pain has lessened. She has had a few urinary tract infections in the past but none in the past 10 years. She had her appendix removed when she was 15 years old and this was an uncomplicated operation for confirmed appendicitis. She lives with her three children on a local council estate. The patient has not been in a long-term relationship since her husband died. However she has very recently started a new relationship and they have been using condoms.

Examination

The GP first assesses her overall well-being. She is not in shock: her pulse and blood pressure are normal (for her) and she has warm and dry extremities and is in no distress. Her temperature is normal. A gentle abdominal examination shows tenderness in the right iliac fossa with no guarding and no rebound. The introduction of the speculum to take some swabs does cause some pain in the lower abdomen and vaginal examination is not carried out.

 INVESTIGATIONS

Urinalysis shows a trace of protein, one plus of blood and no white blood cells or nitrites. This suggests that there is not a urinary tract infection (UTI) but because of her past history of UTIs the specimen is sent off for culture. Swabs are sent to the laboratory for testing. The urine pregnancy test is positive.

Questions
- What is the differential diagnosis?
- What does the GP do now?

ANSWER

> The main four possible diagnoses in this patient are: an ectopic pregnancy, a UTI, pelvic inflammatory disease and appendicitis (this we can rule out as she has had her appendix removed).

She has not had a previous ectopic pregnancy, which this current history points towards. She is pregnant and pelvic inflammatory disease does increase the likelihood of an ectopic pregnancy. This diagnosis is very important to determine as the consequences of missing it could be very serious indeed with sudden rupture of the fallopian tube and life-threatening haemorrhage into the abdominal cavity.

The GP calls the early pregnancy ultrasound unit and arranges for an urgent scan. The scan confirms a pregnancy in the adnexia with a fetal heartbeat present. Given the symptoms and signs and her complicated past history a laparoscopy is arranged. This confirms an early ectopic pregnancy in the right fallopian tube with no signs of active pelvic inflammatory disease. The patient tells the doctors that she probably does not wish to have another child. The ectopic pregnancy with the fallopian tube is removed and the patient makes an uneventful recovery. The vaginal swabs and mid-stream urine (MSU) results are negative for infection. The GP provides her with the combined oral contraceptive pill that she can use in addition to condoms.

KEY POINTS

- Ectopic pregnancies must not be missed as they can be life-threatening.
- Abdominal and pelvic examination need to be gentle when ectopic pregnancy is suspected.
- Multiple pathologies can occur so a pelvic infection and a UTI are also possible in this case.

CASE 5: ACNE

History

The GP is visited by a young man aged 15 years and his mother. The young man seems very uncomfortable and his mother concerned. The mother leans forward to explain the story. The GP encourages the young man to speak and suggests that it might be helpful for the mother to leave the room. The young man decides that he would like to be alone with his GP and he reassures his mother that he will speak about the problem that they have come about. His mother rather anxiously leaves the room.

The patient explains that he has had mild acne for 2–3 years but recently he has noticed more spots on his face and a few spots on his shoulders. He is not looking forward to summer when he will be wearing swimming trunks and wanting to do without a T-shirt. He also tells the GP that he is very keen on one of the girls in his class at school. She also seems interested in him but he feels self-conscious about his acne and this has got in the way of his developing their friendship. He is embarrassed that he should feel this way as his father has told him that it is only acne and that he will grow out of it. His mother is more understanding as she had acne when she was young and still has some pockmarks on her face. She has told him that it did make her very miserable and she never got treatment as there was none on offer at that time. He has not tried anything for his spots, except for over-the-counter medicines, which have not helped. He is worried that his acne is there because he does not wash enough or because he eats fatty food and likes chocolate. He is a healthy person and enjoys football and goes to the gym. He does shower daily and washes his face morning and evening.

Question

- What does the GP do next?

The GP is tempted to leave it at that and prescribe something for the patient's acne: she still has a number of patients to see before the end of the evening surgery. However, something in the way the young man is telling his story prompts the GP to dig deeper. She very seldom sees this patient although she has known him since he was born. The patient is the eldest of four children. His father is a very successful lawyer and his mother looks after the home. She has seen the GP on a number of occasions with mild depression and the GP knows that it is not easy for her as her husband works long hours and, although not cruel, is very tough on her and her children, expecting a lot of them.

The GP asks how things are going. The patient looks down and hesitates. The GP encourages him by asking about his interests. It transpires that the patient is passionate about Drum 'n' Base music. He often has fights with his dad over this as his dad is a classical musician and is not keen on loud music in the house or the fact that the patient enjoys going out to gigs and often comes home late at night during school time. The young man has not known who to go to for support and he does not want to worry his mother about it. The GP offers to spend some time with him talking through the situation and thinking about what can be done to support him. In the back of her mind the GP is also thinking that she may broach the subject of relationships with this patient as this was mentioned by the young man earlier in the consultation. There may also be the opportunity to talk about the use of recreational drugs and alcohol.

Time is marching on. The consultation has already lasted 15 minutes when it was booked for 10 minutes. The GP needs to draw the consultation to a close. Before she does this she talks with the patient about his acne, explaining that it is hormonal in origin and that more washing and changing his diet will make no difference. They decide to start with a simple topical medication, benzoyl peroxide. The GP asks the patient to come back in 2 weeks. This will probably be too early for any noticeable improvement to the acne but will give them more time to explore the other issues. They book a double appointment at the end of an evening surgery.

 KEY POINTS

- Encourage children and young people to talk through their symptoms, rather than leaving it to their parents.
- A simple presentation from a teenager is an opportunity to explore other issues that may be just as important.
- The beauty of general practice is in the continuity of care that it affords. Use this in dealings with patients.

CASE 6: ANAEMIA

History

A 25-year-old woman returns to her GP for a review of her anaemia. Six weeks ago she joined this surgery having just moved into the area and having just found out that she was pregnant – about 8 weeks gestation at the time of the new patient check. Working full-time in the city and in a hurry to get back to work she intended to postpone her first midwife booking appointment to a later time.

INVESTIGATIONS

Remembering her own pregnancy, the practice nurse had taken blood for a full blood count. The results returned showing a microcytic, hypochromic anaemia (mean corpuscular haemoglobin, MCH, 25.6 pg/cell) with a haemoglobin of 10.2 g/dL. The nurse practitioner had prescribed a course of ferrous sulphate tablets at 200 mg three times daily for 4 weeks and asked for a repeat full blood count when the course of tablets had finished. The repeat full blood count results show a deterioration of the anaemia as below.

Haemoglobin (Hb):	9.8 g/dL
Platelets:	384×10^9/L
White cell count:	8×10^9/L
Erythrocyte count:	6.5×10^{12}/L
MCH:	25.6 pg/cell

The bottom of the report includes the following comments from the haematologist: Antenatal haemoglobinopathy screening result: Hb electrophoresis HbF = 0.7% (0.5–2.2), HbA2 analysis above 3.5% (0.5–3.5). β-Thalassaemia carrier, no evidence of sickle haemoglobin, partner testing should be offered.

Questions
- Why did the iron tablets not help?
- What is the significance of this result?
- Why does the baby's father need testing?
- How might you explain the different reporting of the results for the two full blood counts?

ANSWER

The normal physiological increase in plasma volume in pregnancy causes haemodilution in a pregnant woman and can give an artificially low haemoglobin level. However, haemoglobin levels should not fall below 11.0 g/dL and less than 10.5 g/dL is regarded as abnormal. It was reasonable for the nurse practitioner to assume that a microcytic, hypochromic anaemia in pregnancy is caused by a lack of iron. However, the patient is not iron deficient. β-Thalassaemia carriers are well, but are often slightly anaemic, sharing the features of iron deficiency of microcytosis and hypochromia. The distinguishing element is the erythrocyte count which is reduced with iron deficit, but increased in β-thalassaemia carriers.

Haemoglobinopathies are recessive gene disorders. Carriers are usually well and unaffected or only minimally affected. There are many different forms of haemoglobinopathies. The combination of abnormal and missing haemoglobin chains causes a wide range of phenotypical expressions. The patient is a carrier of a potentially severe genetic disease. Delaying antenatal midwifery care caused her to miss the usual screening at 10 weeks gestation by 4 weeks. Her partner needs urgent testing for haemoglobinopathies in order to estimate the risk to the fetus and decide if further tests are required. If the partner tests positive the couple can be offered fetal testing to determine how the child might be affected, as for the fetus there is a one in two chance of being a carrier of haemoglobinopathy and a one in four chance of being either affected by the disease or free of the genetic disposition. It is important to check the patient's family background, previous knowledge and understanding of the disease. Some ethnic groups have a high carrier rate for the gene and the news would be less likely to come as a complete surprise. However, as the patient is well and potentially completely unaware of her carrier status, care needs to be taken exploring the topic. Ideally, she should have been part of the routine antenatal testing programme allowing the midwife to provide sufficient information to allow the patient to give informed consent for testing. Excluding the possibility that the baby's father is a carrier of a haemoglobinopathy allows everyone to relax.

The different reporting of the results for the two full blood counts could be explained by the fact that it is likely the practice nurse did not provide any clinical details with the first full blood count request. A MCH lower than 27 pg/cell in an antenatal patient triggers testing for haemoglobinopathies. The nurse practitioner will have mentioned pregnancy and the lack of response to iron treatment on the repeat blood test request form.

 KEY POINTS

- Watch out: not all microcytic, hypochromic anaemias are caused by iron deficiency.
- It is important to give all essential clinical details when requesting any test.
- Test results in pregnancy may have a different significance compared with tests for those not pregnant.

History

While working a 2-week locum in a colleague's practice, you are consulted by a middle-aged, middle-class lady whose confident, home-counties accent implies a person not to be trifled with, and who is accustomed to getting her own way. She is moderately dismayed by seeing you instead of her 'old friend Tommy' (i.e. your GP colleague). However, as she needs a repeat prescription, she is willing to continue. Her records show a long list of mixed physical and psychological complaints, including hypertension, osteoporosis, asthma, menopausal symptoms, anxiety and depression. All she wants this time is a further supply of her salbutamol inhaler, and her Valium (she takes 5 mg three times a day). A review of past prescriptions shows she is using approximately two such metered-dose inhalers a month, and she does not seem to have been prescribed any steroids, or had a recent asthma check. She has been on the benzodiazepine for nearly 20 years. She is a non-smoker, and drinks, as she says, 'just socially'; you are not clear how much this means as she will not elucidate.

Examination

She is pleased but surprised when you ask to examine her. Her blood pressure is 155/100 mmHg; her lung fields are clear, but her peak flow rate is reduced at 310 L/minute and, according to her age and height, the wheel nomogram on your desk predicts 475 L/minute.

Questions

- Should you give her the prescriptions?
- Should you change her medication, and if so to what?
- What further enquiry might you make in her case?

ANSWERS

You ask her how long she has had asthma, whether she has had any hospital admissions or treatment with steroids (the records may not always be accurate), and how well she understands the inflammatory nature of the disease. Although she says she has little trouble from it, she admits to a daily (and nightly) cough and to breathlessness on mild exertion, such as climbing stairs. You tell her you are happy to give another prescription for salbutamol, but you would like to improve her control, as she seems to need quite a lot of salbutamol with less than perfect results. She queries this, as 'Tommy' never seemed to think it necessary. You say that recent research does suggest tighter control of her asthma will improve her general well-being, and you would like to try her on inhaled steroids. You are able to persuade her to try beclometasone 200 μg, twice daily, and you ask her to see the practice nurse for a more detailed assessment. You write in the notes to the nurse that you would like the patient to be checked for inhaler technique, and to try using a home peak flow meter.

You discuss briefly with her the problems associated with long-term tranquillizer use. You tell her that you will issue a prescription today, for 2 weeks' supply, and you would like her to return again when your principal returns from holiday, to talk about this issue. You write this in the notes, so that he can prepare to deal with it. And you record the slight uncertainty about her alcohol intake on her notes, for his future reference too.

 KEY POINTS

- Be cautious in changing the established treatment plan of another doctor. It may have been negotiated over a long series of consultations, by a doctor who knows the patient better than you, and you may harm the doctor–patient relationship in the future.
- It is simpler not to start a patient on benzodiazepines than to stop them once they have become addicted. Even the rule of thumb ('1 month withdrawal for every year of usage') can be optimistic, and you may have to accept a compromise treatment plan with the patient.
- Do not try to manage too many problems simultaneously: both you and the patient may become confused. Select the most pressing problem first and deal with the others in due course.

History

The GP is visited by a patient, well known to her, who injured his arm the previous day getting out of his articulated lorry. The patient, who is 30 years old, tells her that, while at work the previous day, he slipped in some oil while getting down from his lorry. He was holding onto the hand grip and pulled heavily, twisting his right arm. He now has pain in his right forearm and finds it painful to lift objects with his right hand.

The patient lives with his wife and their four children, the eldest 6 years old and the youngest just 4 months old. They live in a council house on the local estate. Although not very well off, relying on his income with very little savings, they are a happy family. He works long hours, is helpful around the house and spends lots of time with the children. Often he works through the night, helps get the children to school and nursery and, before he sleeps, looks after the youngest for an hour or two so that his wife can get some rest. His health has generally been good although there is a strong family history of heart disease; his father died from a myocardial infarction in his 60s and his brother has high cholesterol and raised blood pressure, controlled by medication. He comes to the GP once or twice a year to get his blood pressure checked and has annual blood tests to check his blood lipids. So far, these have been normal although occasionally his blood pressure is on the higher side of normal at 130/85 mmHg. He is slightly overweight and has been trying to do a bit more walking and playing football with his sons. He does not smoke and drinks minimal alcohol. He has also been attempting to eat more healthily and not eat snacks and takeaways while working. However, his life is hard and it is not easy for him to stay as healthy as he and the GP would like.

Examination

On examining the patient's arm the GP finds that the patient is tender just distal to the lateral condyle of his humerus and although there is good strength there is marked pain on flexion of his forearm against resistance and pain on resisted wrist extension. There is no evidence of bruising or swelling. The patient's blood pressure is slightly raised at 135/87 mmHg. His body mass index is 27.

Questions
- What would the GP be thinking at this stage?
- What immediate treatment could the GP suggest?
- How might the GP deal with this problem in the longer term?

ANSWER

The GP suspects a muscle tear and is very concerned as this man's family depend heavily on him. They cannot afford for him to be off work for too long. However, he should not be driving a heavy truck unless he is physically in good health and an arm injury prevents him from driving safely. The GP is aware that these types of injury can take some time to resolve. Even if he is not working, having to help round the house and look after small children may not give his arm the rest required to heal. The GP is also concerned about other aspects of the patient's health: the patient is at risk of depression, further weight gain and an increase in blood pressure if there is an extended period of inactivity and anxiety.

The GP advises his patient to rest his arm for the next couple of days, supplying him with a sling, and asks the patient to then resume gentle exercise. She also suggests that he apply ice packs for 20 minutes three times a day for the next 24 hours. Because there is no swelling she does not recommend compression or elevation. The GP prescribes a course of oral non-steroidal anti-inflammatory drugs (NSAIDs) having first checked that the patient does not suffer from asthma or indigestion.

The GP tells the patient that he needs to take the ten days off in the first instance and makes another appointment in a week's time. The doctor fills out a Med 3 for the patient to send to his employer to cover this period. She talks to the patient about the importance of not driving until his arm is back to full strength and about sick pay; it appears that the patient should receive this as he has taken only a few days off work in the previous year. However, the GP does ask the patient to talk with his work to clarify his entitlements. The GP makes an urgent referral to physiotherapy for assessment and treatment. As the normal waiting time for physiotherapy is 8 weeks the GP rings and talks with the local physiotherapy department to explain the situation and expedite the process, and manages to get an appointment for the patient at the end of the week. The GP is also thinking that she may need to refer the patient to a rheumatologist or orthopaedic surgeon if physiotherapy does not help.

 KEY POINTS

- Seemingly minor injuries can be more serious and long term than initially thought and may need to be treated quite aggressively from the beginning.
- Treating the patient in their social context is vital.
- The GP needs to think ahead about possible eventualities and plan with the patient accordingly, without unduly worrying the patient.
- The safety of the community is paramount when it comes to driving heavy vehicles.

CASE 9: ARM PAIN

History

The GP is visited by a woman well known to the surgery. She is 60 years old and has a history of hypertension and depression. She is complaining of left arm pain that has been present for a few weeks. She finds it hard to describe the pain and appears very distressed by its severity. She tells the GP that it is a burning type of pain that involves the whole arm from her shoulder to her wrist. Her arm also feels very hot and is particularly sore at night, preventing her from sleeping properly. At times she thinks that her left arm appears swollen and the skin mottled in colour. Moving her shoulder, elbow and wrist joints is painful. Any touch to the skin of her arm is excruciating and she has taken to putting a soft cotton, long-sleeved vest under her clothes to prevent the harshness of her woollen cardigans rubbing against her arm. Six months previously she had fractured her left wrist when she tripped over a low wall in the park exercising her dog. Her wrist had been in a plaster for 6 weeks and the fracture had healed well. She tells the GP that she has not hurt her arm since the fracture and that she holds her dog lead with her right arm. Her dog is small and does not pull on the lead unduly. She has not had a rash or any symptoms suggestive of shingles. Her neck is sometimes a bit sore and stiff but is not a major problem and she has not had any neck injury.

The patient lives with her husband with whom she has had a troublesome relationship. She has few friends and feels lonely and isolated. She has had counselling from the practice psychotherapist and has tried courses of antidepressants but they have not helped very much. She tends to present with many seemingly minor symptoms. Recently, the GP has been concerned that she is drinking too much alcohol. She reports that she drinks red wine at a level of about 20 units per week although recently she sometimes drinks more, especially when she is alone. The GP is perplexed by the pain as it does not fit with anything the GP recognizes or has seen before.

Examination

The GP does a full examination. The arm is exquisitely painful to touch, even with very light touch and these sensory signs do not correspond to a dermatome or to a peripheral nerve distribution. Tone and power are normal as are the reflexes. The skin appears warm and moist compared with that of the right arm. Other than this examination of other systems is normal.

INVESTIGATIONS
Blood tests show no sign of diabetes, liver or renal dysfunction; autoantibody screen and full blood count is normal; and there is no folic acid, iron or vitamin B_{12} deficiency.

Questions
- What could the pain be?
- What might the GP do next?

ANSWER

!

There are a number of possibilities for diagnosis including: simple muscular strain; epicondylitis; brachial or ulnar neuritis (perhaps post-herpetic pain); shoulder pathology; cervical or thoracic disc prolapse or spondylitis; arthritis; thoracic outlet syndrome; angina; malignancy; reflex sympathetic dystrophy; multiple sclerosis; peripheral neuropathy caused by diseases such as diabetes or autoimmune disease.

The GP makes a referral to the local pain clinic and they agree to see the patient urgently. Computed tomography (CT) and magnetic resonance imaging (MRI) scans of brain and spine show no abnormality. Nerve conduction studies are normal. A bone scan reveals increased blood flow to the left arm compared with the right and in view of her history and symptoms a diagnosis of reflex sympathetic dystrophy or complex regional pain syndrome type I is made. This is a complex and poorly understood condition that can occur spontaneously or can be the result of trauma. She is put on gabapentin which does help and nerve blocks are also effective. A course of physiotherapy is instigated. Ongoing psychotherapeutic support is provided. She is also referred to the local alcohol liaison team for counselling about her non-dependent alcohol problem.

 KEY POINTS

- A GP can feel overwhelmed by a patient who is presenting with a symptom where there is not an obvious diagnosis. This does not mean that the symptom is not real or that the patient is not suffering.
- Diagnosis can be especially difficult where a patient is suffering from a number of physical and psychological problems. In this situation a referral to a generalist service, such as the pain clinic, will help.
- Multiple diagnoses require a multidisciplinary approach and the GP has a central role in organizing, monitoring and integrating care.

CASE 10: ARM SWELLING

History

The GP is consulted by a 20-year-old woman with a 2-day history of a feeling of slight swelling and tenderness of her dominant right arm from axilla to fingers. Otherwise she feels very well and has not had any previous illness of note. She has never suffered from anything like this before and would not ordinarily come to the GP with something like this except that the swelling appears to be getting worse and she is concerned about its cause. Her arm does not feel hot and she has not noticed any skin infection or rash. She does not feel feverish and has no other swelling. There has been no trauma. She has just come back from a long weekend camping holiday with her friends. She did not carry a heavy pack as they transported their camping equipment into the camp site by car. They had a quiet weekend relaxing and going for a few gentle walks. They did drink some alcohol and they also smoked a little cannabis but did not take any other drugs; in particular, she does not inject.

She smokes five cigarettes a day and drinks up to 20 units of alcohol per week. She is on a monophasic combined oral contraceptive pill of standard strength and has been on this for 4 years with no adverse effects. She is not allergic to anything that she knows of, although she sometimes suffers from hay fever in the early spring for which she takes an antihistamine. She is at university, studying economics and politics, and lives in a flat with other students. She is a vegetarian and exercises by cycling and walking. She is of normal weight. She has been to see her present GP previously for contraception and was once seen at the surgery with a chest infection. Both her parents are alive and well, as are her two siblings (both are younger than her). There are no particular family illnesses although her paternal grandmother has Type 2 diabetes.

Examination

The GP examines the arm and compares it with her left arm, measuring the biceps and forearm diameters at a fixed distance from the lateral epicondyle. The right hand is slightly mottled. On measurement the right arm is marginally larger than the left although it is her dominant arm. There is no sign of infection or rash, the patient is afebrile and there are no dilated veins on the arm or chest. However, there is some tenderness in the axilla and the axillary vein appears slightly knotty. There is no fullness in the supraclavicular fossa and no lymphadenopathy. The patient's jugular venous pressure (JVP) is not raised and cardiorespiratory examination is normal. The arm is fully mobile but the pain in the axilla is worse with movement of the arm.

Questions
- What is the differential diagnosis?
- What does the GP do next?

ANSWER

> The most common causes of this type of symptom in a woman of this age who is otherwise healthy would be superficial phlebitis, cellulitis, localized allergy, or swelling as a result of trauma. Other causes such as a cervical rib, axillary vein thrombosis, lymphoedema, superior vena caval obstruction or an occult fracture would be unlikely.

The GP is not sure what the diagnosis is and is slightly concerned that there may be an axillary vein thrombosis and so rings the local vascular surgical registrar and arranges for an urgent assessment. A venogram is carried out and it does indeed reveal an axillary vein thrombosis. A thrombophilia screen is negative and the cause is unknown. The patient is hospitalized in the high-dependency unit and warfarinized. This has a good effect, opening up her axillary veins. She continues on warfarin for 3 months and stops the oral contraceptive and smoking. She also reports to the GP that she has stopped drinking alcohol. A follow-up consultation 6 months later reveals that she is well with warm, well-perfused and non-distended veins.

 KEY POINTS

- Although 'common things occur commonly' the unusual can happen and the GP needs to be aware that the unexpected may occur.
- With experience, the doctor becomes increasingly aware of symptoms and signs that, in the context of what they know about the patient, do not fit the normal pattern.
- Whenever you feel unease about a diagnosis or a patient's condition do not hesitate to get another opinion from a colleague in your practice or hospital.

CASE 11: BACK PAIN

History

An 83-year-old man is sent to you with back pain by the nurse who has seen him for a new patient check. She noted that he also complains about tiring more easily and this, together with the back pain, makes standing longer than 1 minute uncomfortable. He tells you that over the last 3 years he has lost power in his legs making it difficult to get up out of a chair or climb the stairs and that he has become unsteady when walking. On questioning he reveals that he is passing urine more frequently, having to get up more often at night time. He admits that the urinary flow is reduced and he feels he has not emptied his bladder completely at times. He has tried to deal with the urinary frequency at night by reducing his fluid intake in the evenings. He has not been to his doctor for years. His only past medical history is an emergency appendectomy age 13. He is a white Londoner, a widower who lives alone in his family home but with good support from his son and daughter and their families who live nearby. The nurse had ordered some routine blood tests as she noted his blood pressure to be elevated at 187/96 mmHg.

Examination

Neurological examination of his legs shows a proximal muscle weakness making it difficult for him to rise from the chair without using his arms. There is no sensory loss and the reflexes are equal in both legs. He has a good range of movement in his spine, but some tenderness over the paravertebral muscles of his lumbar spine. Rectal examination shows a good sphincter tonus, smooth rectal mucosa and an asymmetrically enlarged prostate gland. His blood pressure is elevated at 178/92 mmHg.

🔍 INVESTIGATIONS	
Serum sodium:	150 mmol/L (normal 135–147 mmol/L)
Serum potassium:	3.3 mmol/L (normal 3.5–5.0 mmol/L)
Serum urea level:	9.0 mmol/L (normal 2.1–7.1 mmol/L)
Serum creatinine:	107 μmol/L (normal 62–106 μmol/L)
Estimated glomerular filtration rate (GFR):	57 mL/minute/1.73 m^2 (normal GFR is approximately 100 mL/minute/1.73 m^2 for a white patient who is not a child or pregnant)
Serum calcium:	2.2 mmol/L (normal 2.05–2.55 mmol/L)
Alkaline phosphatase:	56 IU/L (normal 40–130 IU/L)

Questions
- What would your problem list be?
- What is the differential diagnosis?
- Which essential tests would you like to order and in which order?

ANSWER

Your problem list would include back pain with muscle weakness; raised blood pressure readings; urinary outflow obstruction; and hypokalaemia, hypernatraemia and reduced kidney function.

!

A differential diagnosis includes:
- Prostate cancer. This must be considered in any man of his age presenting with back pain and urinary symptoms. The asymmetrically enlarged prostate might indicate a malignant growth within the prostate. The raised blood pressure readings and abnormal blood tests are not explained by this diagnosis.
- Essential hypertension and benign prostate hypertrophy. Both are common diagnoses in elderly men. This patient had not been to his doctor for years making an earlier pickup of the conditions unlikely.
- Conn's syndrome might be causing secondary hypertension in this gentleman. His symptoms of muscular weakness, polyuria and the hypokalaemia on his blood test would all fit with this diagnosis.

In terms of further investigation, prostate-specific antigen (PSA) testing is essential. A normal PSA allows you to start treating his benign prostatic hypertrophy, while a raised test result would indicate a referral to a specialist. An X-ray of his lumbar spine is also essential. Even with a normal PSA and normal serum calcium and alkaline phosphatase it is prudent to exclude any metastatic spread to the lumbar spine in a gentleman of his age. More blood pressure readings are needed to make the diagnosis of hypertension. Home self-monitoring or a 24-hour blood pressure can be helpful in this situation. Repeat renal function tests are needed. A persistent hypokalaemia would be an indication for a 24-hour urinary aldosterone and/or plasma renin and aldosterone measurements.

 KEY POINTS

- Elderly patients often present late in their illnesses.
- Patients who have not visited their doctor for years might have several undiagnosed disease processes going on at the same time.
- Common diseases are common and rare diseases are rare.

CASE 12: BACK PAIN

History

The GP is visited by a 55-year-old woman who has had a 1-week history of lower back pain and stiffness. The pain is deep and aching with occasional sharp and stabbing pains and goes into her buttock and down the outside of her right leg and calf to her right foot. There is some numbness and tingling on the top of her right foot. She remembers a clicking, tearing feeling in her lower back when she bent down to put her shoes on, the day before the pain started. Before that she had been working very hard at her computer and had done a couple of long car journeys to visit her mother who had not been well. The pain is affecting her sleep and is particularly bad in the mornings when she wakes up, making it extremely difficult to get out of bed. She has been unable to sit for any period of time. She cannot stand fully upright. The pain is slightly easier when she is moving and worse when she is still. Other than that, hot showers ease the symptoms temporarily but no particular movements or positions help and the pain makes her very restless. She has been continuing to work but is very difficult to concentrate. She tries not to visit her GP unless it is absolutely necessary but this time feels very disabled by the pain and asks for some stronger pain relief.

She has had a long history of back problems that originated from a swimming accident when she was 16 years old when she was thrown backwards by a wave. She remembers a severe pain in her lower back, feeling faint and having to lie on the beach for some time before the pain and faintness subsided enough for her to go home. The pain lasted for some weeks but she did not see a doctor or seek any treatment. Over the years she has had a few episodes of lower back pain. The pain usually goes down the outside of her right leg to her calf. She has found that moving helps the pain and that, with gentle walks and the help of non-steroidal anti-inflammatory drugs (NSAIDs) and paracetamol, the pain subsides after a few weeks. Once the initial pain has reduced she usually goes to her osteopath and finds that this also helps.

Other than her back pain she has not had any other illnesses of note and is not on any medication. She walks a lot and swims twice a week, eats healthily and is of normal weight. The patient lives on her own and works as a successful freelance journalist. Over the past week friends and family have been popping by and bringing in food and groceries.

Questions
- What questions would be important for the GP to ask?
- What would the GP need to check for in the examination?
- What are the management options?

ANSWER

The symptoms, given the woman's past history, are suggestive of acute lumbar disc herniation on a background of chronic disc pathology. The most important questions for the GP to ask are for red-flag symptoms. If any of these were present then immediate referral would be necessary. The GP should ask about any sensory loss in the buttocks, genitalia or perineum (saddle sensory disturbance), any sphincter disturbance of bladder or bowel such as incontinence or urinary retention, any sexual dysfunction, progressive weakness or bilateral symptoms, and follow up the questioning with an examination that looks for these features, suggestive of the cauda equina syndrome. The findings need to be clearly documented in the notes. Urgent surgical spinal decompression is indicated for these patients to prevent permanent neurological damage.

Examination includes inspection and palpation as well as assessment of movement and neurological testing. A lack of ability to rise from a squatting position suggests an L4 defect, lack of ability to walk on heels an L5 problem and inability to walk on tip-toes an S1 problem; reduced knee jerk suggests an L3/L4 problem and reduced ankle jerk an L5/S1 problem. Sensation to pinprick should be tested for in each of the dermatomes. Straight leg raising and the femoral stretch test are also helpful in diagnosing whether sciatic nerve pain is present.

In this case the symptoms and signs suggest an L5 lesion with no complications. The GP suggests time off work and gentle exercise and prescribes co-dydramol for the pain. Because it has been an ongoing problem the GP decides to refer her and writes to the local orthopaedic surgeon. Unfortunately, the local orthopaedic surgeon does not deal with disc problems and writes back to the GP to say this and suggest a neurological referral. In the meantime the patient develops foot drop. The neurologist responds to say that surgery is not indicated. The patient gets a second opinion privately from another orthopaedic surgeon. She undergoes a discectomy that relieves her pain but unfortunately the foot drop is permanent. The GP has made a serious mistake by referring her to the wrong specialist and then not following this up with ongoing assessment of the patient and an urgent referral to the right specialist.

 KEY POINTS

- Uncomplicated lumbar disc herniation usually settles with pain relief, time and reassurance.
- Watch out for red-flag symptoms that require urgent referral for neurosurgery.
- Follow progress and referrals carefully to prevent grave sequelae such as in this case.

History

An 80-year-old retired school teacher comes to see you. You have been treating her mild hypertension for years with a beta-blocker and a diuretic. She is a frail spinster of the old school, always neatly turned out, and deferring to the doctor in all matters. You inherited her case from your predecessor when you joined the practice some years ago, and she frequently refers fondly to old Dr Jones' skills.

Today, she has come because of a cough which has troubled her for a couple of weeks. It is non-productive, but keeps her awake. You already know she is a non-smoker. She thinks she may have lost weight recently, but complains of no other symptoms. She would like some of the cough mixture which Dr Jones used to prescribe, and which she always found so effective. The computerized records do not reveal it, but searching through her old paper Lloyd-George envelope, you find he gave her 'Mist. Ipecac. et Amm.', which you are surprised to see still listed in the latest *British National Formulary* (BNF) as ammonia and ipecacuanha mixture.

Examination

You ask to examine her. She nods in agreement, removes her coat, and unbuttons the top of her blouse. You ask if she could remove the blouse, so that you can examine the chest properly. 'Oh, but Dr Jones never did that', she declares. You explain that you think it necessary this time, in order properly to diagnose her case; you ask her if she would like the nurse to come in as a chaperone. She says that is not necessary, but only reluctantly removes the blouse. You then see that she has padded out the right side of her bra with a cotton-wool dressing. You ask her to remove this, which she does again reluctantly, to reveal a large fungating frank carcinoma of the right breast.

Under direct questioning, she admits this has been present for some months, but she has been too embarrassed and frightened to mention it. It is not as painful as you might have expected, and she thought it would go away by itself. You ask her gently if she knows what it is, and she says quite candidly, 'Yes, it's cancer, my sister died of it 20 years ago.'

Questions

- What action would you take now?
- Who, apart from a consultant surgeon, would you like to involve in her case?
- How do you diplomatically explain that your management may differ from a colleague's?

ANSWER

You complete the examination, checking the other breast, the glands and elsewhere for signs of metastases. You do not forget to sound her chest, which reveals some basal rales. You explain that you agree with her guess, and even though it is late you think some treatment would make her more comfortable, and may prolong her life. You discuss surgery, radiotherapy and chemotherapy with her, and she agrees to attend the hospital clinic. You immediately fax an Urgent Referral Form to the Breast Unit. You also ask if she would like the community (district) nurse to help her with dressings, and suggest that the local palliative team nurse be contacted for support. Finally, you offer her some antibiotic for her chest infection, explaining that nowadays this is thought more effective than 'Mist. Ipecac. and Amm.', which she can have as well. You ask her to see you after her hospital appointment, to discuss the specialist's advice.

🔑 KEY POINTS

- Resist the temptation to chastise patients for failing to attend earlier. We must offer medical care when the patient chooses to ask for it, not when we think it would do most good.
- When a patient is likely to face intense, high-technology medical care, they are most in need of humane, person-to-person support. The GP is often the best person to provide this, and you will need to keep in close touch with events.
- Do not upset the patient's trust in the profession by deriding a colleague's previous care, unless you think other patients may be at risk from this.

History

The GP is consulted by a patient that he knows well, a 70-year-old woman with a long history of hypertension, mild to moderate chronic obstructive airways disease and generalized osteoarthritis. She tends to get two or three chest infections a year that require antibiotics and steroid tablets. The patient does take her medication but is unable to completely stop smoking even though she has attended the smoking cessation clinic on a couple of occasions. She has smoked for the past 50 years and has recently reduced her smoking from 20 cigarettes a day to two or three cigarettes a day that she smokes outside. She lives with her ailing husband who has dementia, and has a lot of support from her family and from social services. The patient reports that over the past month or so she has found it more difficult to walk up the hill to her house and has been coughing more frequently, even though she has not had any recent chest infections. She also feels very tired. She tells her GP that her breathlessness is only a problem when she walks up the hill, especially in a cold wind. It does not wake her at night. She has some white sputum in the mornings, perhaps a little more than usual. She is not getting chest pain or palpitations, has had no noticeable weight loss, no pain apart from her usual arthritic pain and no ankle swelling. She is not suffering from a change in bowel habit. Things are very stressful at home as her husband is deteriorating and she feels that she cannot cope much longer. She is very sad about this as she would like to look after her husband to the end if it were possible. However, he is up a lot at night wandering and she is worried about leaving him alone for any period. As much as carers and her family help, it is she that carries the burden. She is taking amlodipine, inhaled salmeterol and beclometasone, and paracetamol.

Examination

On examining the patient the GP finds no cyanosis, no clubbing, a normal pulse, a blood pressure (BP) of 140/88 mmHg, no raised jugular venous pressure (JVP), no lymphadenopathy and no ankle or sacral oedema. Her chest has reduced breath sounds generally, as is usual for her, a few early inspiratory crackles and no other abnormal sounds. Her heart does not appear enlarged and her heart sounds are normal. Her abdomen reveals normal liver, spleen and kidneys. Breast examination is normal. Her weight is 1 kg less than 6 months previously with a body mass index of 24. A brief neurological and musculoskeletal examination is normal. The PHQ-9 (see Table in Case 62) depression score is 14 revealing moderate depression and the score is greater than the last time it was done 6 months previously when it was 9 (mild depression score).

Questions

- What would the GP be thinking about as possible diagnoses?
- What examination is important?
- Given the findings what investigations would be helpful?

ANSWER

> The GP would be considering a worsening of her chronic obstructive pulmonary disease (COPD), anaemia, lung cancer, heart failure, thyroid dysfunction and depression as the most likely possible diagnoses. She may have more than one diagnosis.

The GP orders some blood tests that include a full blood count, lipid, liver, renal and thyroid function. He also considers testing for B-type natriuretic peptide (BNP). At that time the BNP is a new test so the GP has to look up the information that he received recently from the local hospital laboratory. He discovers that heart failure is unlikely if levels of BNP are low or normal in an untreated person and so he decides that this is a good test to order. The patient has not had a chest X-ray for 5 years and so he orders one, in particular to make sure that there is no malignancy, as well as referring her for repeat lung function tests that were last done 15 months previously and showed mild to moderate COPD.

The blood test results are essentially normal with no sign of thyroid dysfunction or heart failure. The chest X-ray reveals some hyperinflation but no other abnormality. Her lung function tests have deteriorated somewhat and she now has moderate COPD with a forced expiratory volume in 1 second (FEV_1) of 45% of the predicted value; no improvement is seen post-bronchodilator.

The GP is looking at diagnoses of deteriorating COPD and depression. He ensures that she is taking her inhalers correctly, prescribes inhaled tiotropium instead of salmeterol and beclometasone and refers her for pulmonary rehabilitation. He has found that pulmonary rehabilitation has been extremely effective for other patients. He talks with her about the absolute need to stop smoking and she agrees to go again to the smoking cessation clinic and this time to stop smoking altogether. He organizes for another assessment to be made of her husband's dementia and makes a follow-up appointment with his patient for 2 weeks hence.

KEY POINTS

- As part of every doctor's duty to provide a good standard of practice and care, professional knowledge and skills must be kept up to date.
- As well as good diagnostic ability one of the major skills of an effective GP is the ability to help patients with practical solutions and support for health-related and social problems.
- With health-promotion interventions, deteriorating health can persuade patients to finally make necessary lifestyle changes such as smoking cessation.

History

On a cold February day you are on call, and pick up the phone to hear someone breathing heavily, at first unable to speak. You recognise the breathing pattern as that of a 79-year-old retired council workman, a widower, who has been variously diagnosed in the past with chronic bronchitis, asthma and more recently chronic obstructive pulmonary disease (COPD). He just calls it a chesty cough. You tell him you will call round, but first you check his records, especially his current medication. This includes salbutamol, beclometasone and ipratropium inhalers, theophylline and prednisolone tablets, and over the years an assortment of antibiotics, cough suppressants and expectorants. His last course of amoxicillin was just 2 weeks ago.

When you visit you are admitted by his daughter, who lives nearby. The patient is lying propped up in bed, with a nasal cannula delivering oxygen from the adjoining concentrator. He is a thin man, with an over-expanded chest; his breathing is laboured, his lips are blue-ish, and when speaking he pauses for breath every few words. He says he didn't really improve from his last course of antibiotics, and he is coughing more than usual. He does get out of bed for a few hours each day, and you notice the cigarette stubbed out in an ashtray filled with greenish mucus. His chest sounds as noisy as ever, but there are no local signs of consolidation. He asks for a different antibiotic, but declines any suggestion of being admitted to hospital.

Questions
- How do you arrange oxygen therapy for a patient?
- Is another course of antibiotic indicated?
- How can you discourage him from smoking?

ANSWER

Oxygen is not a panacea for patients with impaired lung function. Pure oxygen is of course toxic, and even a slight increase in inhaled oxygen can reduce the respiratory drive, actually worsening the condition. The patient will have had his lung function assessment done at a previous visit to the Chest Clinic, his blood oxygen and carbon dioxide levels measured, and his response to added oxygen monitored. The Chest Physician is then in a position to tell the GP whether oxygen therapy is indicated, what delivery method (nasal cannulae, or a 24 per cent or 28 per cent face mask – remember, air contains 21 per cent oxygen) – what flow rate is recommended (generally between 1–2 L/minute if using nasal cannulae) and how many hours a day the oxygen should be administered (the closer to 24 hours the better with a minimum of 16 hours). Cylinders are easy to supply, but if the patient needs more than 8 hours a day of oxygen, it is more economical to prescribe a concentrator. This is ordered on a Home Oxygen Order Form and installed by the approved supplier (details are given in section 3.6 of the *British National Formulary*).

Although most respiratory tract infections are viral, this man's chronically damaged respiratory mucosa can offer little resistance to bacterial invasion. It is unrealistic to wait for the result of a sputum culture (though still useful to request it, for future reference), and a chest X-ray is unrealistic unless he changes his mind about admission. Assuming resistance to amoxicillin, you could try a macrolide (e.g. azithromycin or clarithromycin), a tetracycline (e.g. doxycycline), or a quinolone (e.g. ciprofloxacin).

If the disability caused by his restricted lung function, the previous adjurations of you or his other doctors, the nagging by his late wife and his daughter, or the threat of instant immolation owing to the fire hazard of oxygen, have not cured him of his intense nicotine addiction by now, you probably will not be able to get him to desist. He is past the aid of the Smoking Cessation Clinic. He may agree to nicotine replacement therapy, or bupropion, but you may have to accept that he will continue smoking until he dies. It would be honest to say so to him, and warn him and his daughter that he is likely to die, if not from this illness, then from some future exacerbation. However, they probably already know that.

 KEY POINTS

- Remember the old aphorism: 'to cure sometimes, to relieve often, to comfort always'. An incurable, and perhaps untreatable, patient still merits your attendance, support and comfort, even if you can think of little to say. The patient and their family will be grateful, perhaps even more so than those who are readily cured with a simple treatment.
- Cultivate your local specialists, who will appreciate your interest in their field, and will be glad to share responsibility for clinical care in difficult cases.

History

A 58-year-old woman comes to the surgery complaining that her tongue has gone brown, her mouth has been feeling dry and she has been experiencing a bad taste. She has tried a mouthwash and sucking on peppermints to relieve the symptoms. Yesterday, her husband had returned home after a 9-month stint in the Merchant Navy. He has complained that she has bad breath and is disgusted by her discoloured tongue and the patient bemoans that 'now he won't even kiss me anymore'.

The patient is well-known to the surgery. She has a past medical history of depression and attends regularly with chest infections. She suffers from chronic obstructive pulmonary disease (COPD) after 40 pack-years of smoking. Her last infective COPD exacerbation was protracted, needing a second course of antibiotic treatment 2 weeks ago.

Examination

Examination of her mouth shows brown discoloration of her tongue mainly at the base, sparing the tip and the underside of the tongue (see illustration below). The tongue appears furred and it seems as if there are small hairs protruding from the brown discoloured areas. Her dental status is poor with one-third of her teeth missing and widespread and advanced caries in the remaining teeth.

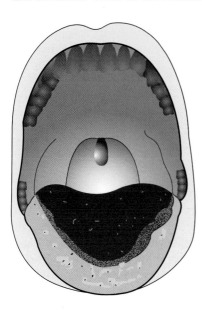

Fig. 16.1 Brown tongue (illustration courtesy of Jutta Warbruck).

After the examination the woman breaks into tears: 'I can't go on like this. I hardly see my husband and now he is rejecting me. I am afraid he might be having an affair'.

Questions
- What is the list of problems?
- How would you treat the brown tongue?
- How would you advise this woman?

ANSWER

Black hairy tongue (lingua villosa) is a harmless condition caused by defective desquamation of filiform papillae of unknown aetiology. Elderly and infirm patients, smokers, tea and coffee drinkers, patients with a poor diet or poor dental hygiene, and patients on antibiotic treatment are more likely to become affected. Addressing the underlying cause often brings improvement. Stopping antibiotics frequently leads to a spontaneous resolution. Increasing the amount of roughage in the diet helps to prevent a recurrence of the condition. One suggested treatment for hairy tongue is to slice pineapples thinly and suck the slices for 40 seconds followed by chewing and swallowing them and to do this for 8 minutes twice daily. After 7–10 days the tongue usually returns to normal.

It is common for seamen to find it difficult to adjust to 'normal' life when returning to their family after long spells at sea and this can result in relationship problems. If problems persist, relationship counselling can be helpful. Some husbands prefer to escape back to work at sea rather than engage in talking therapies.

This patient already suffers from low self-esteem and recurrent depression. In her anxiety she creates new problems by suspecting her husband of having an affair. Smoking-induced lung disease and her tooth decay are strong indicators of a long history of physical self-neglect. Her low self-esteem makes her an unlikely candidate to respond positively to health-promotion messages. Health professionals will have urged her to stop smoking on several occasions and her repeated failure to succeed will have produced a feeling that she has let herself and others down. In this situation it is important to start with easy wins. A trip to the dentist might be more easily achieved than the cessation of smoking. Counselling and cognitive therapy can be helpful to address her negative thoughts.

The episode of hairy black tongue and its probable relationship to antibiotic use is likely to have a permanent shift of attitude toward the use of antibiotics for this woman. While up to now antibiotic treatment might have been an easy fix for her smoking-related disease, she will be more reluctant to use this medication in the future, increasing her motivation to stop smoking.

The woman needs strong reassurance and she can be told that her brown tongue is a harmless condition. In her case there is a good chance that her hairy tongue will improve spontaneously as her antibiotic treatment finishes. The GP can suggest that she talk with her husband and address the problems that they experience readjusting to 'normal' life. The patient can be offered review in a week or two to see if the tongue has returned to normal, whether the relationship problems have eased and whether her mood has stabilized.

 KEY POINTS

- At times minor acute conditions upset patients much more than more serious chronic conditions with insidious onset.
- It is important to consider a patient's emotional ability to respond positively to lifestyle advice.

CASE 17: CERVICAL SMEAR REQUEST

History

The practice nurse storms in to the GP consulting room between patients. She is very upset: 'I have just spent 30 minutes with someone who demands to have an unnecessary cervical smear. She is not eligible to have another test. We already have the results of normal cervical smears taken annually over the last 7 years. I told her so, but she won't listen. I have asked the receptionists to give her your next "emergency" appointment to sort her out. I can't deal with her anymore and I am already running late due to her inappropriate request'.

The patient is demanding to see a gynaecologist. She cannot understand why she has to go to a GP surgery to get her care. She used to live in the USA where she had access to 'proper specialist care'. Her gynaecologist did her smear annually explaining to her how important it was to detect cancer early.

The GP asks her to sit down so that he can take a history before they make any decisions. The patient is a mathematics professor specializing in statistics. She is 33 years old and has been married for 10 years to a fellow statistician. She has no history of sexually transmitted infections, had four sexual partners before marriage and states that she has never had sex outside marriage. Her periods are monthly, lasting for about 3 days and she does not have any intermenstrual bleeding. Her husband uses condoms for contraception. She does not like the additional risks related to the pill; neither does she like the idea of an intrauterine device. She is a non-smoker. None of her relatives died or suffered from cancer-related illnesses.

Having taken a history the GP informs her that her risk of developing cervical cancer is very low and that she is next due for her smear in 2 years' time as part of the national screening programme for cervical cancer. The patient gets very upset 'All my friends at home have their tests done annually. Are you trying to tell me they got this wrong? When the nurse told me the same story a year ago I did my research. I figured out that the relative risk reduction of having annual tests compared to 3-yearly tests is statistically significant. You are just trying to save money for the NHS. I have two small children that I want to see growing up. I want to avoid all risks possible. Please, can't you just do the test for me?'

Questions
- What options does the GP have in response to the patient's request for a smear test?
- Why do GP and patient disagree about the risk of developing cervical cancer?
- Is the frequency of smear tests in the NHS national cervical screening programme reduced because of its cost?

ANSWER

Principally, the GP can either agree or refuse to do the test. However, ideally, he has the time and skill to negotiate a mutually agreeable solution to this problem. When the nurse refused the patient's request for a cervical smear, communication broke down. It might be tempting just to do the test and get on with normal business but one of the functions of the GP is to be the official gate-keeper for NHS resources. As correctly identified by the practice nurse, the patient has no indication for this test. If the GP breaks the rules by sending a test he is also undermining the nurse. The GP could offer the patient a private gynaecological referral or a self-referral to one of the private health-check providers. The GP has to be careful not to give the impression that the test is needed and that the patient has to pay for it because of rationing of NHS resources. Arranging tests for anxious patients is unlikely to reduce anxiety for long. The converse often happens: patient anxiety increases by acknowledging patient's irrational concerns as appropriate. If the outcome is a private referral, a well-written referral letter to the gynaecologist allowing the specialist to appreciate the situation makes it more likely that she/he will back up the GP's and nurse's message.

The GP is talking about the patient's absolute risk of developing cervical cancer. He noticed the absence of all risk factors and the previous normal test results. The point at which low risk becomes medium or high risk is based on scientific evidence and expert opinion. The patient talks about relative risk. Relative risks can sound quite dramatic when used outside their context and doubling of risk can sound very worrying. The doctor's role is to communicate risk in context.

Any screening programme aims to maximize benefits and minimize harm and cost. Through statistical modelling, experts have worked out that it is safe to offer cervical smears at certain intervals. Patients at risk, for example those with mild dyskaryosis, are offered more frequent testing. Possibly, more frequent testing for all is likely cause harm: women will be inconvenienced having to take time out to undergo the tests; the number of false positive tests will increase proportionally with the number of tests conducted, resulting in unnecessary fear and investigations; and the money spent doing these test will not be available to provide other services.

 KEY POINTS

- Patients may perceive themselves to be at risk of potential disease at a different level from that perceived by health professionals.
- Patient estimation of their vulnerability to illnesses can be higher or lower than estimations based on medical science.
- A patient's perceived risk is often based on their illness perception. This patient fearing cervical cancer will perceive herself to be more vulnerable if she is frightened about developing the disease.

CASE 18: CHEST PAIN

History

Your next patient is a worrier. He is a 48-year-old shopkeeper, originally from Sri Lanka, with a wife who is the business head in the family, a teenage daughter who is studying A-levels and on track to become a doctor, and a merry younger son who delivers your morning paper. This patient is a frequent attendee at the surgery, with minor complaints. Today he describes pain in the chest, which has been coming and going for about 6 months. He feels it in the front of the chest, on the left side, and is able to pin-point it with his finger. He does not associate it with normal activity or with meals, and it does not wake him at night (though he sleeps poorly, he says). He eats a balanced diet, thanks to his wife's good sense, and he is spare rather than fat; he is a non-smoker, and drinks only rarely. He has in the past been offered a variety of treatments, including anxiolytics and antidepressants, but at present takes no formal medication. He does not find paracetamol or ibuprofen makes much difference to his pain.

He has a family history of heart disease. His father died in his 60s, of a heart attack. He has an elder brother in Sri Lanka with angina. His mother is in her 80s, and has diabetes.

Questions

- What further questions might you like to ask him?
- What causes of chest pain occur to you, and what occur to the patient?
- How much examination and investigation is appropriate here?

ANSWER

Like most differential diagnoses, the causes of chest pain can be thought of as a two-by-two matrix: serious or not serious, likely or not likely. It is mandatory, in a middle-aged man, to consider coronary artery disease, which is likely to be in his mind already. You might also think, with decreasing probability, of pleurisy, pericarditis, a mediastinal tumour or an aortic aneurysm. The long timescale, and the absence of developing serious signs, point to a simple explanation: intercostal muscle pain, perhaps a forgotten minor injury leading to a bruised rib, possibly reflux oesophagitis. Problems such as a pulmonary embolus, or a viral myalgia such as Bornholm's disease, would have a more acute course.

Simple examination reveals no signs of heart disease; his blood pressure (BP) is merely 135/85 mmHg, his pulse rate 84 beats/minute. You ask for fasting lipids and glucose, a blood count and erythrocyte sedimentation rate (ESR), a chest X-ray, a resting and an exercise electrocardiogram (ECG), all of which return normal results. At this point a cardiovascular cause seems unlikely. Symptomatic treatment, such as a topical non-steroidal cream, may relieve his pain. If he remains anxious, especially regarding his family history, you may discuss the merits of seeking a second opinion, though more detailed cardiac investigation can be uncomfortably intrusive.

His chest pain, though now demonstrably non-serious, remains a mystery, until you visit his shop to pay your paper-bill. There you see him unpacking heavy parcels of newspapers, lifting them manually onto the shelves. Musculoskeletal pain in the intercostals seems a natural consequence, and an informal chat over the till serves to relieve his anxiety for the time being.

KEY POINTS

- When puzzled by a set of symptoms, try to structure your approach: here in terms of relative importance, or by system (musculoskeletal, cardiovascular, etc.) or by aetiology (traumatic, infective, etc.)
- Your working diagnosis may be unclear, and you will often have to make management decisions based on probabilities rather than certainties. Be prepared to adjust your ideas if new facts appear, as in this case, serendipitously.

CASE 19: CHEST PAIN

History

You see a 27-year-old man, an office manager in a design studio in London, who does not have much of a past medical history. For the last 3 days, he has been experiencing sharp, stabbing and burning pain in his right side, just under the rib-cage. He does not remember injuring himself and self-treatment with pain-killers (paracetamol and ibuprofen) and with antacids (Gaviscon and ranitidine) have had no effect. The pain is bad enough to wake him at night.

His record reveals several episodes of mild anxiety, sometimes treated with benzodiazepines or latterly serotonin-type antidepressants, but none of them long-lasting or requiring hospital care.

Examination

On examination, you find a slim, healthy-looking man with no obvious signs except some hypersensitivity around the right costal margin. His liver is not palpable, and there is no increase in pain on inspiration. His lung fields are clear. His facial expression is slightly drawn, and he admits the pain has been quite bad: on a scale of one to 10, he puts it rather precisely at 8.

Questions

- What likely explanations are there for his pain?
- How might the illness develop over the next few days?
- What treatments are available?
- What further questions or investigations might you consider?

ANSWER

Biliary colic is possible, but he is young, slim and male, which make it less likely. The absence of adventitial lung sounds makes pleurisy also unlikely. It could be a simple musculoskeletal pain, caused by an unnoticed injury, but the nature of the pain is not typical. Alternatively, he could have the prodromal symptom of a zoster infection – pre-herpetic neuralgia, involving dorsal root 9 or 10. Indeed, he develops a red, blistery rash over the painful region in the next few days, just as you warned him to expect. The pain is severe and persistent, requiring time off work.

Even before the rash appears, as you are confident of the diagnosis, you offer him specific antiviral medication: aciclovir tablets, 800 mg, taken five times a day (breakfast, lunch, tea, supper, bed-time) for a week. A brisk analgesic, such as diclofenac or co-dydramol, is necessary. After the rash fades, there is some post-herpetic neuralgia, and you add in amitriptyline for this neuropathic pain. Gabapentin is an alternative, and sometimes the topical application of capsaicin cream helps, or lidocaine-medicated plasters.

Herpes zoster is a late consequence of childhood chickenpox, and is usually seen in the elderly, or in those whose natural immunity is impaired perhaps through a recent illness such as influenza. It is unusual in a young, fit man, and you ask if there is any possibility of him having a lowered immunity. He reveals that he is homosexual, with a long-term partner. Over the time that they have been together there is no history of other sexual relationships for either partner. Nonetheless, you counsel him that a *Human immunodeficiency virus* (HIV) test might be indicated here, noting that the consequences of a positive result can have profound effects on him and his relationship: probably a reduced life expectancy, the need for permanent therapy, the avoidance of all unprotected sex in future depending on his partner's HIV status, even the probability that he will not be able to get life insurance.

 KEY POINTS

- Illnesses in general practice often present early, before a complete diagnosis is feasible. It is worth being aware of the prodromal phase of illnesses, as accurate prediction of the natural history is, historically, one of the skills of a doctor.
- The same aetiology can have widely different consequences at different ages. Herpes zoster infection is hazardous to the fetus and pregnant mother, mostly harmless to school children and unpleasant and wearisome to the adult, in whom it can also be a flag for other problems.
- This man is gay: however, do not be influenced by the stereotypical notion of the 'gay man with HIV'. Any person in front of you may have HIV.

CASE 20: CHEST PAIN

History

You are consulted by a 22-year-old single man, just graduated and working in a pub-lishing office. He has a past history of asthma and currently uses a salbutamol inhaler intermittently. His presenting complaint is of chest pain: for the last month or so, he has been experiencing localized, left-sided pain in his ribs, which he indicates with his fingers 'just here', pointing to ribs 5–8 in the anterior axillary line. The pain is rather sharp, lasts up to 5 minutes, and does not seem to be related to anything he is doing at the time. He is a non-smoker, drinks a glass or two of wine or some spirits, not every day, and lives at home with his widowed mother. The pain does not last long enough to be worth taking pain-killers. He is concerned, because his father died a few years ago of a heart attack.

Examination

Examination reveals a thin young man, slightly anxious, with a pulse of 92 beats/minute, blood pressure (BP) 110/50 mmHg, normal heart size and sounds, and clear lungs. His ribs are not tender to touch, or on 'springing'. His peak flow rate is 580 L/minute, which is normal for his age and height. He is not particularly athletic, but does play occasional weekend football.

Questions
- What possible diagnoses might you consider?
- What investigations are appropriate?
- What can you advise him about these symptoms?

ANSWER

The history does not suggest angina, although this is clearly in the back of his mind. The most likely cause is simple musculoskeletal pain, caused by some unnoticed strain, not resolving quickly because it is impossible to rest the rib muscles. Less likely causes might be a small pneumothorax, costochondritis (Tietze's syndrome), Bornholm's disease (especially if there have been several cases locally), or pre-herpetic neuralgia. All of these are unlikely given the intermittent and somewhat prolonged course of the disorder.

The main theme will be to establish good rapport, so that the patient has confidence in the benign nature of the diagnosis. Although you may be reasonably confident of this on the history alone, it is important to take his anxiety seriously and not immediately 'reassure' him there is nothing wrong. The very act of examining him is helpful. Too much investigation at this stage might reinforce his anxiety. You may want to offer simple analgesia: an anti-inflammatory such as ibuprofen, either orally or in this case perhaps topically – it is said to have more than just placebo value – and suggest that he returns in a week or two, to review progress.

If his symptoms persist, some basic tests could be done: an electrocardiogram (ECG) would be prudent, a chest X-ray is possible, and in view of his family history a blood test for lipids would help. If the tests are clear, as is likely, he can expect to recover spontaneously in a few weeks, but you could emphasize the need for 6-monthly asthma checks with the practice nurse for as long as he needs the salbutamol.

 KEY POINTS

- Since common things occur commonly, the simplest diagnosis is often the right one.
- Anxiety (whether patient's or doctor's) about missing a serious but rare illness should be dealt with rationally, by the traditional methods of history, examination and investigation.
- A large part of the art of medicine is knowing when to stop investigating.

History

A 52-year-old businessman attends the emergency surgery at his general practice with a 3-hour history of right-sided chest pain. The pain developed suddenly when he stretched to pick something up from the ground in the office. It is a sharp stabbing pain, made worse by deep breathing, but is not related to any movements. He denies any feeling of breathlessness. He had a previous episode of chest pain 3 years ago, which was diagnosed as acid reflux and which responded well to treatment with a proton pump inhibitor. He stopped smoking 10 years ago, but previous to that he smoked socially, up to 10 cigarettes a day, for 25 years. He has noticed that he has been sweating more over the last 6 months. He has otherwise been healthy although he works hard and does not eat well or get enough exercise.

Examination

On examination there is no chest wall tenderness, percussion shows hyper-resonant sounds over the right lower chest, and auscultation reveals diminished breath sounds in the right anterior lower chest area. He is profusely sweating, but his temperature is 36.8°C. He has no lymphadenopathy. His oxygen saturation on air, measured with a pulse oximeter, is 98 per cent. His body mass index is 28.5.

Questions

- What is the diagnosis?
- Are there any complications associated with the condition?
- What is your management plan?
- When do you follow this patient up?
- The repeat chest X-ray, taken 1 week after the event, has been reported as normal. Does this finding change your diagnosis or management plan?

ANSWER

The man has suffered a spontaneous pneumothorax. The history of smoking is a predisposing factor. The incidence is about 2 in 10000 with a recurrence rate of about one in ten. However, the sweating remains unexplained. Tension pneumothorax causes acute progressive shortness of breath with positive pressure in the pneumothorax inhibiting venous return and cardiac output: it is an emergency and needs immediate treatment by drainage; however, most spontaneous pneumothoraces resolve without intervention. The history of this patient excluded a tension pneumothorax and he was safe to return home. Patients suffering from mild breathlessness or continuing to be troubled by pain should be seen in casualty to have an X-ray early. Needle aspiration of the pneumothorax can accelerate recovery since the spontaneous absorption rate is only 1–2 per cent of volume per day. The patient was advised about analgesia.

A further chest X-ray after 7–10 days should show complete resolution. The history of sweating needs further investigations, including full blood count, erythrocyte sedimentation rate (ESR), glucose and thyroid function tests. The chest X-ray should exclude tuberculosis as the reason for the night-sweats. The fasting glucose test showed 6.5mmol/L indicating impaired fasting glycaemia, giving a possible explanation for the newly developed sweating. The abnormal blood glucose value needs to be followed up as a routine appointment. Discussions about weight loss and a healthy lifestyle are in order. The patient needs clear instructions that the development of breathlessness constitutes an acute emergency.

 KEY POINTS

- Patients' presenting signs and symptoms might not always tie up nicely to one diagnosis.
- It is important to keep an open mind for unexplained signs and symptoms, which might portray a secondary diagnosis and/or a developing disease process.
- Doctors have the opportunity to follow up patients using time as a diagnostic tool.

History

The next patient is 6 weeks old, and has been brought to the health visitor's routine Child Development Clinic for examination. He is the first-born of his Ghanaian parents; his father is a banker and his mother is a former nurse. His mother had a normal pregnancy and delivery, and is comfortably breast-feeding him.

He is robustly healthy, with no signs of congenital disease or developmental delay. His length and weight are consistently on the 75th centile. He has no heart murmurs, normal hips and genitalia, and good reflexes. You discuss immunization with his mother, who is very willing for this to be done. While she is re-dressing him, she asks if he could be circumcised, like all the other males of her tribal community.

Questions
- What would be your response to this question?
- To whom can you refer for further advice?

ANSWER

The usual reasons for childhood circumcision are: hypospadias (when it is often part of a longer series of operations); abnormality of the prepuce (e.g. phimosis), obstructing the flow of urine; religious custom (e.g. Jews and Moslems); tribal custom (as in this case); hygiene (requested by parents).

The consensus of medical opinion in the UK is that routine circumcision of a healthy boy is not indicated. The anaesthetic and surgical risks, slight as they are, are not justified by any supposed benefits to 'hygiene'. As a result, circumcision without clinical need is not available through the NHS. Many paediatric urologists will carry out such a procedure at the parents' request privately, using local or, in older children, general anaesthesia.

Circumcision for religious reasons can be carried out by medical or non-medical persons, both of whom usually undergo a long programme of training for this procedure. Such operations may also be offered to those outside the religious groups. You may not directly refer patients to non-medically qualified persons for surgical treatment, but it would be reasonable to advise the parents to contact the authorities at the local synagogue or mosque for a list of approved and trained circumcisers.

The postoperative care is normally carried out by the person doing the operation. If a child is brought to you for advice afterwards, be prepared for the operation site to look granular for a week or so. Sutures are not used outside hospital practice. Infection is rare, and antibiotics are seldom needed. Of course, if there is a history of bleeding disorder, the parents should be warned not to proceed with circumcision. If there is a religious issue, they may wish to discuss it with, for example, their rabbi or imam.

 KEY POINTS

- Over the years, medical opinion has varied between enthusiastic support for, and virulent opposition to, routine circumcision. Although you must give your considered opinion, always respect the views of the parents in such a case.
- Female circumcision, however, is a seriously mutilating procedure, and is illegal in this country and many others. If you suspect this may occur to your patient, you should take legal advice on what steps to follow.

History

The warden of one of the local sheltered housing establishments calls the GP to report that one of the residents is not well. When he checked on her in the morning she appeared dishevelled, agitated and confused, and he noticed lipstick smeared over her face and on the mirror in her room. Her niece also rings the GP and is very concerned as she has just visited her aunt having being rung by the warden and has never known her like this before. Your patient is 87 years old and is normally a quiet and digni-fied resident, seemingly contented, and has never behaved like this before. She lives alone and has been a resident there for 7 years. She has one son who lives and works in Singapore and this niece who lives close by and keeps an eye on her. Her health has generally been good apart from a nasty bout of shingles the previous year with post-herpetic neuralgia. This was treated with a small dose of gabapentin and settled after about 6 months. She does have osteoarthritis of both knees, which affects her mobility. Paracetamol keeps the worst of the pain at bay, especially at night. However, she is unable to walk far on her own except around her house, and depends on her niece to take her out in the car which she does most weekends. She is a retired school teacher and is a keen reader and enjoys Radio 4. Blood tests and examination 3 months previously were normal. She has a carer who does her laundry, cleans and shops for her. She has had input from occupational therapy and physiotherapy and her flat is adapted so that she can cook and look after herself otherwise.

Examination

On examination, in particular of the cardiovascular and neurological system, no abnor-mality is found. She is unable to answer the Folstein's mini-mental state examination as she is confused, bewildered and disorientated in time, place and person. There is no sign of any injury. She is afebrile and she does not have respiratory symptoms.

	INVESTIGATIONS
	It is not possible to take a urine sample or do a urinalysis at this time. Urgent blood tests are taken to check full blood count, urea and electrolytes, blood sugar, liver function, thyroid function and calcium and phosphate levels. All blood tests are normal apart from a slight neutrophilia and a mildly raised erythrocyte sedimentation rate (ESR).

Questions

- What is the differential diagnosis of acute confusion in an elderly woman?
- What elements of history, examination and investigation would help in this case?
- What does the GP do now?

ANSWER

Confusion can be caused by delirium, dementia, major depression or psychosis. In this situation the patient's decline has been rapid and she has been well leading up to this illness. The GP is therefore looking at the diagnosis of delirium. The most common causes of delirium in this situation are medication or an intercurrent illness such as infection, head injury, a stroke or a metabolic disorder.

The GP is unable to take a history from the patient as she is too confused to cooperate. However, the warden, the carer and the niece help piece the story together. The patient has been fine up until a couple of days before when she seemed a little confused and not as active as usual. The previous weekend she had had a very happy outing to the local picture gallery. On looking around her flat no medication can be found except for paracetamol. She no longer has gabapentin prescribed and the niece tells you that she got rid of the extra gabapentin when the medication was stopped. No-one is aware of her having fallen or complained of any particular symptom. The carer has, however, noticed that the patient has had an odd fishy smell recently and has been incontinent of urine on a couple of occasions, which is not usual. She is not sure that the lady drinks enough as she often finds half empty cups of cold tea in the flat.

A urinary tract infection is the most likely diagnosis. No-one is keen to move the patient out of her flat for additional care as this will only disorientate her further. They decide to treat her with trimethoprim on the assumption that this is a urinary tract infection, most likely caused by *Escherichia coli*. The carer stays to clean up the flat and wash her dirtied clothes and the niece offers to stay with her aunt through the day and make sure she drinks enough fluids and takes her antibiotics. The warden agrees to drop in regularly and check on progress and the GP tells them that she will ring back in the afternoon to see how things are. The patient is much better by the evening but because delirium is often worse at night, her niece decides to stay the night. By the next day she is starting to regain her equanimity. Once the course of antibiotics is completed a mid-stream urine is collected and this is clear of infection. The niece, carer, warden and patient herself agree to keep a close eye on early signs of a repeat of this episode and the patient agrees to increase her fluid intake.

 KEY POINTS

- In an elderly woman with acute confusion always think of a urinary tract infection as a possible cause.
- Sometimes collection of a urine sample is not possible and the illness has to be treated without a firm diagnosis.
- Other causes must not be ruled out and a close watch must be kept on progress.

History

The GP is asked to call on an 89-year-old widow, who has lived in her own bungalow since her husband died a few years ago. She has Type II diabetes, controlled with diet and metformin, and is handicapped by gradually worsening macular degeneration. Her memory for recent events is faulty, and she has fallen once or twice, on one occasion fracturing her pelvis which necessitated admission to hospital and a painful recovery. It is becoming clear to her daughter, if not to herself, that she is finding it difficult to care for herself, even with a daily home help. She has finally been persuaded to move in to her daughter's home, which has been adapted to offer a convenient 'granny flat' on the ground floor. You are asked to visit her, as she has had 'a funny turn' and cannot seem to speak. Her daughter says she was well on waking, but became confused while being helped to the toilet and seems unable to stand unaided – she normally walks with a Zimmer frame.

Examination

She is sitting in a chair, looking a little puzzled. She is unable to give a history, answering just 'yes' to any question. She seems to be unwilling to use her arms or legs, although there is no evidence of pain or injury. There are no clear lateralizing neurological signs. Her pulse is 86 beats/minute, somewhat irregular, and her blood pressure is 125/65 mmHg – rather low for her. She has no carotid bruits.

Questions

- What diagnoses should you consider?
- What are your options for her further care?
- What investigations might be helpful?

ANSWER

!

On a background of probable vascular dementia, she may have had a non-paralytic stroke. Her possible atrial fibrillation may have triggered a small thrombus into the brain. If the symptoms clear within 24 hours, it would be classified as a transient ischaemic attack (TIA). Or she could have a diabetic problem: hypo- or hyper-glycaemia. Or her confusion might be a non-specific indicator of an occult urinary tract or respiratory infection.

Using her glucose meter, you check her blood glucose and it is 6.7 mmol/L. You test the urine in her commode with a multistrip and this shows a trace of protein, some glucose, but no nitrites, leucocytes or blood. While this is going on she makes a gratifying recovery. She asks for a cup of tea, recognizes and begins to converse with her daughter and you, and after an interval is able to get up with assistance and walk a little with her frame.

You explain to them that you think she has had a TIA. She is at risk of further episodes, and might suffer a full stroke. She could be admitted to hospital for more detailed investigation, such as a computed tomography (CT) scan, but she is reluctant to leave her comfortable home; her daughter is willing to continue caring for her and will monitor her progress. You would also consider a full workup for atrial fibrillation: ideally, this would require anticoagulation but in view of the danger of bleeding with warfarin given the history of frequent falls you decide to just add a prescription for aspirin and dipyridamole to her medication. You agree to revisit the next day, and arrange a care programme with the Community Team. Her Abbreviated Mental Test Score, measured later, is only 3 (where out of 10, 8 or more is normal and 7 or less significant). After discussion with her daughter you decide at this point not to refer her to a clinic to assess the use of a cholinesterase-inhibitor. The patient lives contentedly on for a further 2 years, before dying peacefully of a stroke at the age of 91.

KEY POINTS

- Full investigation of a probable stroke would require admission, but the logistics of this can be formidable for frail elderly patients: being taken out of familiar surroundings, away from the family, being shaken about in an ambulance, being interrogated, undressed, punctured and intubated by kindly but strange uniformed staff, can be profoundly disturbing experiences.
- Step back from the acute diagnosis and assess what is in the best interests of the whole patient.
- Using time to establish the natural history of an event is one of the most valuable resources for the GP.

CASE 25: CONFUSION

History

A 60-year-old woman asks her GP to visit. She lives alone on the third floor of an apartment building in a well-kept privately-owned flat. Her friend lets the GP in as the patient is feeling too shaky to come to the door. She reports that she woke the previous night to go to the toilet, felt confused, lost her way and fell in the kitchen. She thinks that she momentarily lost consciousness, but managed to crawl to the toilet and get back into bed. In the morning she woke to find blood on her pillow case and on her nightdress. She called her neighbour who reports that she found her a little confused, which is unusual as she is normally very alert in the morning. She is a head-hunter in a large and busy city recruitment agency and works long hours, thoroughly enjoying her job. She is not looking to retire for at least another 5 years. She is a long-term patient at the practice but does not come very often as she feels healthy. The last time that she was seen was 1 year earlier when she presented with a sore back as a result of an overenthusiastic weekend gardening spree. Her blood pressure, weight and general examination at that time was normal and her back settled over a week with rest, non-steroidal anti-inflammatory drugs (NSAIDs) and private physiotherapy that she had access to through her company. Since then she had been in good health and is not on any medication. She eats sensibly and walks in the country most weekends with her friends, being a member of a local rambling club. She has not smoked for over 25 years and enjoys a good red wine, drinking about 12 units per week and never more than two medium glasses (4 units) at a time as she feels uncomfortably tipsy on more than this. A recent check-up at work revealed a non-fasting total blood cholesterol of 4.2 mmol/L and a random blood glucose of 5 mmol/L, both normal. She has not had any serious illness and her parents are both still alive in their late 80s, frail but otherwise well.

Questions
- What does the GP need to explore in the focused history and in the examination?
- What is the differential diagnosis?

ANSWER

The GP asks the patient about her health in the weeks leading up to this episode. She reports that she has not been feeling very well in the last few weeks – not like her normal self. She has noticed that her concentration has not been as good as usual, has had a slight frontal headache and has been feeling a bit nauseated and dizzy. These symptoms are at their worse when she wakes up and improve during the day. She has not had a fever, dysuria or frequency. The GP specifically asks her whether, apart from the night before, she has had any falls or head injuries recently but she has not. On examination the GP notices that she has bitten her tongue and that she has bruises on her left arm and a small cut on her left knee. She is of good colour and her respiratory, cardiac and neurological examination is normal. She is afebrile and urinalysis is normal.

The differential diagnosis in acute confusion includes hypoxia, systemic infection, cerebrovascular accident, hypoglycaemia, diabetic ketoacidosis, alcohol withdrawal or intoxication, electrolyte imbalance, uraemia, effect of drug or medication, myxoedema, cerebral tumour, post-ictal state or carbon monoxide poisoning.

The GP goes through some of these diagnoses and the patient's history and examination findings do not fit. However, very fortunately for the patient, a few weeks earlier another patient had told the GP that she had had her yearly gas fire check by the council and that they had found a gas leak. This patient had been feeling headachy, sick and sleepy for some time and felt herself lucky to be alive. The GP would not normally have thought of this diagnosis but because of the other patient's experience suggests that the patient have her gas-fired boiler checked immediately, and stay with her neighbour until this is done. As a result, a gas leak is found and the boiler repaired. Her symptoms disappear with no recurrence of the confusion. The patient installs carbon monoxide monitors on both floors of her apartment.

 KEY POINTS

- Carbon monoxide poisoning kills 50 people and seriously injures nearly 200 in the UK each year. The overwhelming majority of cases go unrecognized, unreported and untreated.
- The symptoms of carbon monoxide poisoning are like many in general practice: subtle and easy to miss but once diagnosed, never forgotten.

History

The GP has been helping to look after a patient with Parkinson's disease (see Case 95), who was diagnosed with the condition 1 year earlier. The patient has been visiting the Parkinson's Clinic regularly and has been on Sinemet for 1 year and is now on Sinemet plus. He is still playing bowls and going on holidays but is finding that he is sleepy and tired, and getting more forgetful. He is also having problems with his short-term memory and on two occasions he even got lost in his own house. In addition, he finds that he is having difficulty rolling over in bed and fell out of bed when he was staying with his son in Scotland a few weeks previously. The GP does a simple assessment. The patient scores 9 out of 24 on the Epworth Sleepiness Scale, a negative result in terms of a sleep disorder. On the Folstein's mini-mental state examination he recalled three named objects immediately but only one out of the three at 5 minutes. The patient is unable to read and write properly as the war interrupted his studies so the rest of the test is difficult. However, he can draw the intersecting pentagons and obey the three stage command. He did, however, have difficulty with repeating 'No ifs, ands or buts'. The results are suggestive of cognitive impairment.

Questions

- What does the GP do next?
- What other health-care and social-care practitioners would be of assistance in this situation?

ANSWER

The GP refers the patient back to the Parkinson's Clinic and the specialist makes no change to his medication but refers him for neuropsychometry for assessment. He also refers him for some physiotherapy. He sees him again in 6 months and the patient reports that he is now feeling uncomfortable is bed, claustrophobic and hot and is getting out of bed up to 10 times in 1 hour. This is a problem for both him and his wife as getting in and out of bed is difficult. As a result, neither of them is getting much sleep. His hand tremor is also getting worse. Unfortunately, he did not go for neuropsychometry as he felt embarrassed to do so. The specialist suspects that he is actually going 'off' in bed and adds some more Sinemet last thing at night. He also encourages him to continue with the physiotherapy as this is helpful and go for his neuropsychometry testing.

He is seen again 6 months later when the patient reports hallucinations when he sees familiar people and animals that have passed away some years previously. He still has not gone for his testing and is not keen to do so and so this is shelved. The specialists explain to him and his wife that his hallucinations and confusion may be caused by dementia with Lewy bodies. They add entacapone to his Sinemet to try and improve his symptoms at night. Unfortunately, within a few days of starting the entacapone he develops worsening hallucinations and, despite stopping the medication, the hallucinations continue and cause him and his family distress and confusion as he is not sure what is real and what is not. His physical symptoms of Parkinson's are under good control and so the specialist suggests cutting back the Sinemet slowly to see if it is excessive dopamine that is causing the hallucinations. Quetiapine is added for his psychological problems but this has no definite benefit and in fact seems to make him more confused and slow. He is therefore put onto rivastigmine.

The Parkinson's disease nurse specialist and the GP arrange a social service referral and a daily care package is put into effect. The most difficult time for his wife is at night as the patient tends to get out of bed and roam round, and she is worried that he will fall or wander out of the house. A night sitter is arranged for two nights a week so that his wife can have some proper sleep. The patient also is signed up for a day centre.

 KEY POINTS

- Dementia is an extremely difficult condition to deal with and can be frightening and gruelling for the patient (and their carers).
- A multidisciplinary team approach is vital in providing proper treatment and support for the patient and their family.
- Regular follow-up and medication review is essential as symptoms and circumstances can constantly change.

History

A 15-year-old woman attends the evening emergency surgery with her mother. Asked what the problem is her mother starts talking while Emily sits quietly, her gaze down towards the floor. 'I want you to start Emily on the Pill. I have just found out that she is sexually active and at 33 I am not yet ready to become a grandmother!' On further questioning the mother tells you that she found a pregnancy test in the bin and confronted with the object the young woman had admitted that she had used it last week when her period was late. She was relieved to find the test was negative, but she continued worrying. Fortunately, she had started bleeding yesterday.

The GP asks the mother if it would be possible to talk to the patient on her own but meets resistance. 'I have an open relationship with my daughter and we don't have any secrets' she says. 'You wouldn't want me to leave would you?' and the patient nods assent.

The GP informs the patient that the legal age of consent for sexual activity is 16 and that he needs to ask further questions in order to comply with the rules for prescribing contraceptives to underage women. He tells her that it is good that she informs her parents of her activities. He also informs the pair that, once he has satisfied himself that the patient is mature enough to engage in sexual behaviour, he is allowed to see her alone and prescribe contraception. He asks her if she is in a relationship with a man. Mother interrupts 'I know who it is. She has been together with the neighbour's son, since she was nine. He is such a good boy and a good influence on her'. The GP asks the patient what kind of sexual activities she has been engaged in and how often in the last 3 months. 'We did it twice last month' she answers holding her head low. On direct questioning about whether the sexual act involved penetration she murmurs 'mmm'.

Her past medical history reveals no contraindications for the combined oral contraceptive pill. She has no personal or family history of deep vein thrombosis, is not diabetic and has never suffered from focal migraines. Her blood pressure is 124/74 mmHg.

Questions
- What concerns does this scenario raise?
- How should the GP manage the situation?
- What rules govern the provision of contraception to underage women?

ANSWER

This is a difficult situation. The GP has to decide whether it is probable that she has engaged in consensual sexual activity, making a judgment about how the mother's insistence on being present at the consultation has altered her responses. In the majority of cases the situation will be harmless, with the mother simply being protective. However, there is a small chance that the mother does not leave because she is trying to conceal facts that would raise concern about possible sexual abuse. Her presence has made it difficult to determine the consensual nature of the patient's and the neighbour's relationship and to verify that this is her only sexual partner. It is important that young people understand the consensual nature of sexual relationships as they are vulnerable to coercion and peer-group pressure can play an important role in their behaviours. A large age difference between the patient and her sexual partner(s) would be worrisome and below the age of 14 years the authorities view sexual intercourse as child abuse and oblige practitioners to report such situations.

A full sexual history is helpful in tailoring health-promotion advice. The combined oral contraceptive pill offers inadequate protection against sexually transmitted infections and young people are often unaware of the risks involved in varied sexual activities. The patient is clearly engaging in unprotected sexual intercourse and she is at risk of falling pregnant. Starting her on the combined oral contraceptive pill will reduce this risk significantly and she needs to be counselled about safer sex practices. Provision of a short course of the pill would ensure that she returns soon, hopefully to be seen alone; a failure to attend follow-up raises concerns. The local family planning clinic is an alternative for care should she feel uncomfortable with her family GP and a referral letter to the clinic might allow the clinic doctors to keep the GP informed.

The Fraser Rules (formerly known as Gillick competence) govern the provision of contraception to underage women and state that, even without parental knowledge or consent, a doctor or health professional is able to provide contraception, sexual and reproductive health advice and treatment to a young person aged under 16 years, provided that: the young person will understand the professional's advice; the young person cannot be persuaded to inform their parents; the young person is likely to begin, or to continue having, sexual intercourse with or without contraceptive treatment; unless the young person receives contraceptive treatment, their physical or mental health, or both, are likely to suffer; the young person's best interests require them to receive contraceptive advice or treatment with or without parental consent.

 KEY POINTS

- A parent present in the room usually makes it difficult to talk with a young person about their sexual history.
- Counselling about sexually transmitted infections and safer sexual practices is an integral part of consultations about contraception.
- Providing a safe and non-judgmental consultation for the young woman makes effective ongoing care more probable.

History

A 49-year-old air hostess books in to see the GP for her 12-weekly Depo-Provera injection. She usually sees the practice nurse for this procedure, but the nurse is currently on leave. The medical records reveal that the patient has returned for the injections regularly for the last 4 years.

Being unaware of the patient's reasons for this choice of contraceptive method the GP takes a contraceptive history. The woman says that she is very satisfied with her current choice of contraception. She used to rely on the combined oral contraceptive pill (COCP) until the age of 45 years, when she was advised to stop. At the time she was happy to reduce her risk of deep vein thrombosis also having read about the increased risk with flying and changed to the progesterone-only pill (POP, mini-pill). However, because of her international flight schedule, moving daily between time zones, she found it impossible to take the POP reliably at the same time of the day and at the time the newer POP that gave her an increased window of safety was not available. Coming off the COCP her menstrual loss was heavier and lasted two extra days, interfering with work. She returned to see the nurse who started her on the Depo-Provera injection. Initially the woman suffered some irregular and erratic light vaginal bleeding, but since the second injection she has not had any further periods. She is delighted that her monthly bleeds have stopped and she denies any hot sweats or perimenopausal symptoms. She asks the GP how she would know she has reached menopause so that she can stop her injections. The woman has been pregnant once and the pregnancy ended in a miscarriage. The investigations that followed revealed a bicornuate uterus.

The GP is concerned. Recommendations from drug manufacturers include careful re-evaluation of the risks and benefits of treatment in those who wish to continue use for more than 2 years. He knows there have been concerns about loss of bone density associated with administration of the drug. Assessing the woman's risk for osteoporosis extends his history taking.

She has never smoked and drinks less than 3 units of alcohol per week. She eats a balanced diet with at least 1 pint of milk per day and two fish meals per week. Her body mass index has always been around 22. She takes part in sporting activities at least three times a week. In the summer she plays tennis twice a week and goes to aerobic dancing class once a week. In winter she substitutes her tennis with jogging or badminton. The woman is aware of the risks of osteoporosis related to the injections and to her age. She has no family history of osteoporosis and has never broken a bone. The woman is quite clear that she wants to continue with this contraceptive method.

Questions
- What contraceptive options does this woman have?
- How should the GP manage this woman's situation?

ANSWER

Above the age of 45 years the COCP is not recommended and the POP is incompatible with her working schedule. Uterine abnormality is a contraindication to insertion of an intra-uterine contraceptive device (IUCD). Male and female condoms and diaphragms are possible choices for contraception and here one has to take into account accessibility of emergency contraception in case of contraceptive failure.

Once the GP has discussed the alternative contraceptive options it is reasonable for him to continue prescribing the injection. The patient is clear that she wants to continue with this method of contraception; she seems well informed and is able to give informed consent. She has taken all steps to reduce the likelihood of loss of bone density. The evidence about reversibility of bone loss associated with the drug is not clear and no study has proven an increased risk of fractures. However, it is prudent to avoid potential risks wherever possible.

The drug side-effect of amenorrhoea is an important secondary gain for this patient. Being free of monthly bleeds allows her to fit into a working rota easily. Much of the controversy about injectable contraceptive methods comes from the USA where its use has been associated with administration to vulnerable groups without consent, to achieve 'menstrual hygiene' (amenorrhoea). With the contraceptive injection it will not be clear when menopause has begun as menstrual patterns are not normal on the injection and those using the injection do not generally have oestrogen deficiency symptoms. However, follicle-stimulating hormone (FSH) levels can be measured when on progesterone-only medications. It is common practice to stop the injection at the age of 50 years and see if the woman is menopausal. However, if menstruation resumes, the GP will find it difficult to find guidelines on how to proceed with managing her needs. Advice from a family planning practitioner would assist in this situation.

 KEY POINTS

- Choosing appropriate contraceptive methods can be difficult for older women or women in specific occupations.
- Manufacturer's recommendations can put prescribers in a quandary when they conflict with common management practices.

CASE 29: COUGH

History

Your next patient is a florid, plump, forthright woman of 52 years, who is complaining of an irritating cough for the last week or two. She works as a waitress or bartender, and is married with three children. The cough is non-productive and is disturbing her sleep. She admits to getting breathless on climbing stairs, but she is familiar with the symptom and is merely asking for a repeat prescription of her regular cough medicine. The computer records only date back 6 years, so you ask the receptionist to find her old Lloyd George paper records, and in the meantime examine her.

Examination

You note her being overweight, almost obese: she weighs 14 stone (90 kg) and is 5 feet 8 inches tall (175 cm), giving her a body mass index of almost 30. You also note her nicotine-stained fingers: she smokes about 20 cigarettes a day, less now, since the ban on smoking at work. Her throat is slightly inflamed. She has a scattering of coarse rhonchi, but no rales. You guess that she may have a mild exacerbation of chronic obstructive airways disease. Her peak flow rate is certainly reduced (300 L/minute).

The records now reveal that she has been prescribed variously simple linctus, ipecacuanha with morphine linctus and pholcodine linctus by one of your predecessors in the practice.

Questions

- What treatment might you rationally advise?
- What other advice might you offer her?
- What further investigation is appropriate?

ANSWER

Rationally, no treatment at all might be acceptable. Most coughs are self-limiting and generally caused by a viral infection. There is little evidence that expectorants or cough suppressants are helpful; the combination of both in Mist. Ipecac. et Morph. is distinctly unscientific. Your patient can get symptomatic relief by inhaling steam from a bowl of hot water (some people like to add a fragrant oil, such as friar's balsam), from drinking extra fluids and from getting more fresh air. To explain why you are departing from your predecessor's prescription habit, you might say that medical evidence has become clearer since his time, and you would like to offer her the best available modern treatment. The lung findings might suggest you could offer a course of antibiotic.

Of course, you will want to encourage her to stop smoking. You may be able to offer her a leaflet, or arrange an appointment to see the smoking cessation nurse. Her airways may improve with an inhaled bronchodilator such as salbutamol, but she will need careful instruction on how to use it properly. If she does not improve within a month, a chest X-ray is indicated. She will require lung function tests to investigate possible chronic obstructive airways disease. It is also a good idea to check her lipids, and her blood glucose. If you have one available, a carbon monoxide meter can reveal to the patient the extent of harm her smoking is causing. Although she would benefit from losing weight too, you feel this is sufficient for one day and postpone that particular discussion.

 KEY POINTS

- Your advice not to use cough mixture is likely to be received sceptically by the patient.
- Patients can purchase simple cough remedies over the counter, but they are not thought to be any better than nothing at all.
- It is not good practice to decry past inappropriate prescribing as this will likely impair the patient's confidence in you more than in the previous doctor.
- It is more important to gain a patient's trust than to treat everything at once.

History

Gemma, aged 2 years, is brought to see you by her mother, because she has had a cough for about a week. Gemma is a cheerful and active child, who was born after a normal pregnancy, and has had all her immunizations to date. The cough is dry, and tends to keep her awake, which makes her more irritable than usual and she is not her usual bouncy self. There was not much of a prodromal illness.

Examination

On auscultation, you find a localized patch of crepitations in the right mid-lower zone postero-laterally. Her mother asks if she can have a cough mixture to ease the symptom.

You tell her that Gemma has a minor chest infection, and prescribe amoxicillin sugar-free suspension, 250 mg three times a day for a week. She asks you whether Gemma should also have a chest X-ray.

Questions
- What are the likely causes of cough in children?
- What other questions might you ask the mother about this child?
- What investigations and follow-up, if any, would you advise?

ANSWER

The vast majority of childhood coughs are viral in origin, usually an upper respiratory tract infection with post-nasal drip. They tend to resolve spontaneously over 2–3 weeks, regardless of any treatment offered. There is no convincing evidence that cough mixtures, whether placebo, or antihistamine- or decongestant-based, make any difference. The mother may already have discovered this, and you can reinforce the best symptomatic treatment: inhaling steam (by letting a kettle boil in the room – supervised of course – for 10 minutes two or three times a day), fluids, and fresh air.

Remember to inspect the eardrums, as inflammation of otitis media commonly irritates the vagus nerve on its way through the middle ear. Chest infections, suggested in this case by the positive lung findings, can supervene, and are more likely to be caused by a secondary bacterial infection. It is reasonable to offer an antibiotic here. Less commonly, a persistent cough might be caused by whooping cough (although this patient has been immunized there is still a risk, with a recent study showing that nearly two in five children that went to their GP with a persistent cough were found to be suffering from whooping cough). Remember to ask if anyone at home smokes, and if so, ask them to stop.

Has Gemma being eating foods such as peanuts? An inhaled foreign body impacting in the (usually) right bronchus can give a troublesome cough, and if you have such a suspicion a chest X-ray is called for. Otherwise, an X-ray is usually not needed unless the signs and symptoms fail to respond. You might need to explain about avoiding unnecessary radiation, particularly in children.

A follow-up examination next week should reveal a satisfactory resolution of signs, although the symptomatic cough may persist for up to a month or even longer.

 KEY POINTS

- Common things occur commonly, and it is reasonable to assume a simple cause for such an episode.
- If the illness does not follow the straightforward course you predict (Plan A) consider alternatives which may be less common, but more serious (Plan B).
- Remember whooping cough as a common cause of persistent cough, even in immunized children.
- Use antibiotics judiciously, following guidelines such as those from the National Institute for Health and Clinical Excellence (NICE).

CASE 31: DIARRHOEA

History
An 8-month-old baby with diarrhoea is brought to her GP by her mother. Since a holiday visit to Turkey 1 month previously, the baby has had up to four watery loose stools a day. Her mother has also observed that the stools are smellier and paler than usual. Before their holiday she was having one or two soft bowel motions a day. The child is otherwise well and growing normally. She has a healthy appetite and enjoys her food and is active and happy. She was breast-fed up until 6 months of age. She lives with her parents and two older siblings aged 5 years and 7 years in a well-maintained three-bedroom semi-detached house. Her mother works as a part-time teaching assistant in the local primary school and her father is a real-estate agent. The two older children are at school during the day and the baby attends a nursery when her mother is working. The rest of the family are well and have not had diarrhoea; there is no recent history of gastroenteritis in the family or in the nursery.

Examination
A recent growth check shows that she has maintained her weight and length on the 25th centile. On examination there is nothing abnormal to find; in particular her abdomen is soft, non-tender and no masses are felt.

Questions
- What is the diagnosis?
- Which investigations would you order?
- What advice do you give to mother about the child's dietary needs?

ANSWER

This baby has toddler's diarrhoea. The diagnosis of toddler's diarrhoea can be made in a child that is well, grows and plays normally, and is not bothered by the diarrhoea. It is thought that an excess of undigested sugars in the large bowel causes an increase in the water content of the large bowel, resulting in watery motions. As the child grows bigger, the large bowel is thought to become more efficient and the problem resolves. Stool cultures should be taken – two or three samples on different occasions. The recent travel history makes it necessary to exclude bowel pathogens so an examination for ova, cysts and parasites is included.

The mother should be advised about the 'four Fs':

- *Fat*: toddler's diarrhoea is more common in children that eat a low-fat diet. The diet of pre-school children should contain 35–40 per cent fat. Choose full-fat milk in preference to skimmed milk, yoghurts, cheese, milk puddings and other dairy products.
- *Fluid and Fruit juice*: some children drink only fruit juices or squashes to quench their thirst. Mothers should be advised that water is preferable. Fruit juice contains carbohydrates that are not digested or absorbed before the passage into the large bowel. Clear apple juice seems to be the worst in this situation. The sugar in the drinks can spoil a child's appetite leading to a tendency to eat less fat and fibre at normal meal times.
- *Fibre*: children should have plenty of fibre such as fruit, wholemeal bread and vegetables. Fibre absorbs surplus water in the bowel, making stools more bulky and less runny.

 KEY POINTS

- Children differ from adults in their dietary needs.
- Healthy eating advice for children needs to be tailored to their age.
- Reassurance is an important tool in the GP's armamentarium.

History

A 73-year-old man is brought by his wife to the Monday morning emergency surgery. She reports he had 'gone all funny' on Saturday afternoon. When she returned home from shopping her husband was sitting in his armchair having difficulty speaking to her. His words seemed slurred and unclear. His face had changed, with the right side appearing to be motionless. She had problems getting him to bed as his right side seemed to be weak. She had phoned the surgery and was redirected to NHS Direct who suggested she call an ambulance, but he did not want to do that or go to hospital. On Sunday morning the man seemed a lot better having recovered the strength in his legs and arms. His face looked nearly normal and his wife was able to understand most of his speech again. He states that he is back to normal and does not know what all the fuss is about.

Examination

On examination the man seems to be well oriented and his speech is clear. The GP cannot identify any facial weakness. The power in his limbs is normal as is the rest of the neurological examination. His pulse is regular at 78 beats/minute and his blood pressure is 158/95 mmHg. There are no carotid bruits.

The GP reviews his past medical history. The patient rarely attends the surgery and he last came with a chest infection 2 years ago. It was noted then that he was a smoker and he was offered treatment at the nurse-led smoking cessation clinic. His blood pressure was noted to be mildly elevated at 164/92 mmHg. A blood test and a follow-up appointment were arranged, but he had not returned. He has no repeat medications.

Questions
- Was NHS Direct correct in advising acute admission?
- What is the main challenge for the GP in this situation?
- How should the GP manage this patient?

ANSWER

National clinical guidelines from the Royal College of Physicians state that all patients with a transient ischaemic attack (TIA) or a stroke should be admitted to hospital as an emergency with the expectation that they will be managed on a stroke unit. Exceptions may include those relatively few patients for whom the diagnosis will make no difference to management, for example where optimal management is palliative care.

The GP is faced with a patient who is in denial about his health status. He has a long-standing past medical history of raised blood pressure, smoking, and failing to engage with health services. The TIA is an urgent wake up call: the risk of developing a stroke after a hemispheric TIA can be as high as 20 per cent within the first month, with the greatest risk being in the first 72 hours. The GP should refer the patient to a dedicated specialist service as soon as possible, at most within 7 days of the incident. A prompt appointment at the specialist clinic underlines the seriousness of the condition to the patient and helps him in taking his health seriously. This patient's symptoms have resolved and he should be prescribed aspirin at an initial dose of 300 mg daily, continued until a definitive diagnosis and management plan is established. The patient must be warned that should any of his symptoms return within a week he needs emergency admission for immediate investigations.

Patients who have suffered a stroke remain at an increased risk of a further stroke of 30–43 per cent within 5 years. Patients suffering from a TIA or stroke also have an increased risk of myocardial infarction and other vascular events. Transient ischaemic attack and stroke patients should be entered onto the practice chronic illness register and offered systematic assessment of risk factors, interventions to reduce risks, and regular follow-up. This patient needs to have repeated blood pressure measurements. According to the British Hypertension Society guidelines, persisting high blood pressure readings over the next two weeks should be treated with a thiazide diuretic or an angiotensin-converting enzyme (ACE) inhibitor, or preferably a combination of the two. All patients with ischaemic stroke or TIA who are not on anticoagulation should be taking an anti-platelet agent (i.e. low-dose aspirin at 75 mg daily, or clopidogrel, or a combination of low-dose aspirin and dipyridamole). Anticoagulation should be started in every patient with persistent or paroxysmal atrial fibrillation unless contraindicated. Patients with a fasting cholesterol of more 3.5 mmol/L should start treatment with a statin unless contraindicated.

It will be a challenge to engage this patient and help him to adjust lifestyle factors such as stopping smoking, increasing regular exercise, improving his diet to achieve a satisfactory weight, reducing his intake of salt and avoiding excess alcohol.

 KEY POINTS

- Patients' and doctors' assessments of health status might differ widely.
- Acute illness events might allow you to successfully challenge patients' health perceptions.
- A patient with signs of a TIA or a stroke requires urgent referral to a specialist unit (where possible).

CASE 33: DYSPHAGIA

History

A 56-year-old man attends the emergency clinic at his GP surgery. He received a letter giving him an appointment date for his planned upper gastrointestinal endoscopy in 6 months time. He is distressed and tells the GP that he cannot wait that long. His records show that he has experienced worsening indigestion over the last 3 months and that 3 months ago he presented with heartburn that occurred mainly after food and at night. He had had a similar episode 2 years earlier and the GP had arranged a gastroscopy which was normal. At the time he had responded well to a 1-month course of lansoprazole at 30 mg daily. This time his regular GP had started him on lansoprazole, but at a lower dose of 15 mg daily. After 3 weeks symptoms were only partially improving and the GP increased the dose back to 30 mg daily. The patient had then returned, reporting an initial improvement followed by a deterioration that included pain with swallowing. Next the GP had referred him routinely to the open access upper gastrointestinal endoscopy unit.

Now, on further questioning, the GP at the emergency clinic finds out the patient has developed a feeling of food getting stuck behind his breast bone and, as a result, has changed his diet to soft foods to avoid choking. He denies vomiting any blood or melaena.

Examination

On examination he has lost 3 kg in weight, but he does not look unwell. His physical examination is, except for mild epigastric tenderness on palpation of his abdomen, normal.

Questions
- What is the differential diagnosis?
- How would you manage this patient?
- Can you apply the National Institute for Health and Clinical Excellence (NICE) guidelines for patients with dyspepsia here?

ANSWER

Gastro-oesophageal reflux disease might be causing the symptoms and oesophageal stricture is a possible complication. Oesophageal cancer is a rare disease, sometimes developing slowly, either as a result of chronic epithelial damage (Barrett's oesophagus) or spontaneously. The patient is distressed and anxious and, related to this, globus hystericus (a feeling of tightness and of food getting stuck) is a possibility but is usually limited to the throat. However, our patient describes food getting stuck behind the breast bone.

The patient is distressed. He needs to be listened to, his worries explored and the referral chased up. A change of referral status is justified because of the changes in the patient's symptoms that qualify him to be referred under the 2-week rule for suspected cancer. The patient must be informed that the change to an urgent referral status is to investigate him for possible cancer. The real challenge is to communicate the possibility of cancer to the patient without causing undue alarm.

At this stage of the presentation the NICE guidelines can be applied easily. The patient's problem with swallowing food changes the clinical presentation. At the beginning of the consultation the GP will have had problems deciding if the patient's symptoms were part of a 'new' presentation or not, and if the failure to respond to treatment resulted from insufficient dosage of the medication.

Subsequently, the patient is diagnosed with oesophageal cancer. The GP brings this case to the next critical event meeting: could they have done anything differently?

 KEY POINTS

- Guidelines for common presentations in general practice are not always easy to apply. It is not always possible to decide whether the initial patient's presentation is a recurrence of an existing problem or the development of a new problem.
- It is important to keep an open mind and react to changes in the clinical symptoms that patients present.
- Take situations such as this to your clinical meetings in order to share best practice.

CASE 34: ERECTILE DYSFUNCTION

History

A patient attends his surgery for review of the investigations for his erectile dysfunction. He is a 55-year-old fit and muscular landscape gardener who is well known to his GP. Three years ago he was successfully treated for a depressive episode with a 6-month course of antidepressant medication. He describes his relationship with his wife as close and loving. They have always liked to be physically intimate and used to have a regular sex-life. Over the last 2 years he has noticed his erections becoming less strong and more recently he has experienced erectile failures that have become more common. He has not noted any early morning erections in the last few months. He is sexually interested in his wife and he is worried that she is 'missing out'. He denies any relationship problems or symptoms of depression. He stopped smoking 5 years ago after 30 pack-years of smoking. He drinks up to 14 units of alcohol per week, mainly at the weekend. He is not currently on medication.

Examination

On physical examination the GP finds normal external genitalia, with adequate-sized testicles and normal secondary hair distribution for a man. Rectal examination shows a normal-sized prostate with a firm nodule of about 1.5 cm in diameter in the right lobe.

INVESTIGATIONS
The GP orders a serum glucose, full blood count, liver function tests, urea and electrolytes, creatinine, thyroid function tests, serum testosterone, prolactin, luteinizing hormone, sex hormone-binding globulin, and prostate-specific antigen (PSA). The results of the tests are all within the reference range of normal.

Questions

- What is the differential diagnosis?
- What are the next steps in management?
- Which tests/examination did the GP initiate that were not indicated by the patient's initial presentation?
- What further tests might the GP have reasonably ordered?
- What would you tell the patient?

ANSWER

> The differential diagnosis includes primary erectile dysfunction and suspected prostate cancer. The history gives no indication of psycho-sexual problems and he has fully recovered from his previous episode of depression.

All the investigations for secondary causes of erectile dysfunction are normal. About 10 per cent of men between the ages of 40 and 70 years of age suffer from complete erectile dysfunction and his presentation is typical of this. The incidental finding of a small hard nodule in his prostate is unrelated to his initial presentation and requires urgent referral to urology services under the 2-week rule for suspected cancer.

Suspected prostate cancer in a young man needs urgent ultrasound guided transrectal biopsy of the prostate. The histology shows a poorly differentiated adenocarcinoma, Gleason score 8. The patient undergoes a radical prostatectomy 2 weeks later and the postoperative staging shows that his cancer was detected unusually early in Stage 1. The consultant urologist was very happy with the treatment outcome saying 'your GP saved your life by referring you early'.

The patient could be treated with sildenafil for his erectile dysfunction. Primary erectile dysfunction does not meet the NHS eligibility criteria for funding. However, after the radical prostatectomy (with a 50 per cent incidence of impotence) the patient would qualify for NHS treatment.

The guidelines for evaluation of erectile dysfunction do not include a PSA and rectal examination and currently the NHS does not support universal prostate cancer screening of the population. Erectile dysfunction is not a common presentation of prostate cancer. The patient did not have a family history of prostate or breast cancer in first-degree relatives. The patient had not been asked to give informed consent to the additional test and examination and it would be possible to argue that the GP committed assault by doing them.

Patients with primary erectile dysfunction have an elevated risk of developing coronary heart disease and the GP might want to estimate the cardiovascular disease risk in order to initiate treatment if the risk is elevated.

Any prostate lump needs urgent investigations to exclude cancer. Patients who are referred under the 2-week rule must be told that they need to see the specialist for possible cancer. Doctors in secondary care expect patients to know why they have been prioritized for urgent care. Not telling patients that they have signs of suspected cancer can lead to severe communication problems, causing resentment which can complicate future patient treatment.

 KEY POINTS

- Investigations and examinations not indicated by the patient's presenting symptoms need informed consent.
- Occasionally, additional tests uncover severe pathology unrelated to the patient's presentation.

CASE 35: FACIAL PAIN

History

Your next patient is a 55-year-old woman, married with three grown children, who has been experiencing pain in the left side of her face for some months. It is not constant, but can last for an hour or two when it comes; it is severe, throbbing or stabbing in character; and seems to arise in the cheek, radiating down to the side of her jaw and neck. She does not associate it with activity, but finds eating sometimes triggers a spasm. Sometimes her jaw locks and can take minutes to relax. It can last into the night, and is disturbing her sleep. She has not found paracetamol or aspirin helpful. She is a quiet, sensible though somewhat anxious woman who often comes with her husband, an electrical engineer. They are non-smokers and abstemious drinkers, and have little in the way of previous medical history.

Examination

On examination, the left side of her face is slightly sensitive to a gentle tap, but there are no other localizing neurological signs. Her blood pressure is 135/75 mmHg, pulse 88 beats/minute and heart sounds normal.

You suspect trigeminal neuralgia, 'tic douloureux', and prescribe carbamazepine. At first, she gains some relief, but the symptoms break through even with increasing doses. She and her husband are becoming increasingly despondent about this problem.

Questions
- What alternative diagnoses can you suggest?
- What investigations might be appropriate?
- How would you manage her care now?

ANSWER

Her erythrocyte sedimentation rate (ESR), calcium, cholesterol and electrocardiogram (ECG) are all normal. Her temporal mandibular joints are normal on X-ray, and her dentist reports no disease. She becomes disheartened by the lack of progress, and is pleased when you suggest seeking a second opinion from a hospital specialist about her atypical facial pain. Meanwhile, you arrange an ultrasound scan of her face. You treat her with amitriptyline, and gabapentin, and even sometimes with morphine, all of which give temporary relief. The neurologist confirms the original diagnosis. Eventually she is offered partial ablation of the trigeminal nerve which gives her long-lasting relief at the cost of some problems of mouth dribbling and a slight asymmetry of the face.

 KEY POINTS

- When a diagnosis is not immediately obvious, it helps to use a structured plan to differential diagnosis. You might choose a systematic approach (is it cardiac, neurological, vascular, dental, endocrine, psychiatric, and so on?) or diagnose by cause (infectious, malignant, degenerative, immunological, iatrogenic) or by severity (is the patient endangered by possible coronary or malignant disease, or loss of sight?). Each possibility suggests its own line of investigation.
- Some tests can be done in parallel, to save time; some have to be planned serially, to save resources.
- Don't forget, at the heart of this diagnostic puzzle is a woman in misery. Symptomatic treatment is often needed before a final diagnosis is reached.

CASE 36: FAINTNESS

History

Walking past a bus-stop, you see one of your patients, pale and leaning as if feeling faint. She was delivered 6 weeks ago of a son, her fourth child. He was born at home, but the midwife had a difficult time, owing to a brisk and unexpected postpartum haemorrhage. Emergency admission, evacuation of retained products of conception and a three-unit blood transfusion restored the patient to health. You ask her to come to your postnatal clinic that week. Fortunately, the baby is quite unaffected by her faintness, and is thriving: she is breast-feeding him. She now has no problems, apart from tiredness which she expects, having to care for four children. She eats what she describes as a healthy diet, mostly vegetarian but with some chicken, fish and eggs. Despite her parity, she is reasonably slim, and has a fair complexion. Her uterus has involuted satisfactorily, and she has not yet started menstruating. You discuss contraception with her and suggest a low-dose progestogen-only pill.

Examination

You examine her, particularly to assess pulse and blood pressure. Her pulse is 84 beats/ minute and regular and her blood pressure is 110/70 mmHg. When she gets off the couch she feels a little giddy and you have to gently support her to the chair. However she dismisses this as trivial and you can detect no postural drop in blood pressure.

 INVESTIGATIONS

You arrange a full blood count, ferritin, B_{12} and folic acid levels.

Questions

- Does this patient have a problem; if so, what is it?
- What action should you take?

ANSWER

The warnings are there: a haemorrhage, a low-iron diet, tiredness, fainting and a pale complexion. The blood test confirms a low haemoglobin of 7.6 g/dL, with a microcytic picture. Her ferritin level is low, while her B_{12} and folate levels are satisfactory. You discuss with her the merits of another blood transfusion but she is reluctant, partly because she did not like the earlier experience and partly because she does not want to leave her children again. Parenteral iron is unpleasant to receive, and not necessary if she can absorb iron orally. You prescribe ferrous sulphate, 200 mg three times daily, and ask if she can go so far as to adjust her principles and take meat: lamb or beef, once or twice a week. Fresh fruit, with its vitamin C, will enhance her absorption of iron. A blood count 3 weeks later, shows her haemoglobin as 9.8 g/dL, and she is beginning to feel more energetic. You advise a 3-month course of iron and a careful follow-up.

KEY POINTS

- Blood transfusions have a limited life, and anyone anaemic enough to need one should be offered iron afterwards to restore the ferritin reserves, which are depleted by each pregnancy.
- Once haemoglobin concentration and red cell indices are normal continue iron treatment for 3 months to replenish iron stores.
- A follow-up blood count after a few weeks could have detected this problem. Think ahead!

CASE 37: FALLS

History

An 83-year-old man returns for review of his treatment. Three weeks ago he had fallen in his living room late at night and, being unable to get up, he had spent the night on the floor where his wife had found him in the morning. He had been taken to the Accident and Emergency Department of the local hospital by ambulance but, as no fracture had been found, he had been discharged home, the GP being told the next day. At the time he had complained to the GP of stiffness and pain in the muscles of his shoulders and pelvis, his neck and lower back. Further questioning revealed a long, slow decline of energy over the last year. His wife complained that her husband seemed to have lost interest in his surroundings, sitting in his chair reading or watching television all day. 'He used to be so much of an outdoor man' she says. Systematic enquiry uncovered a history of low-grade sweats and long-standing cough (this he had been told to expect by his previous GP after 60 years of smoking).

Examination

The muscles were found to be tender to palpation and he was seen to have problems rising from a chair, needing to rock back and forth using his arms to push his weight upwards.

🔍 INVESTIGATIONS

The GP had arranged the following tests: erythrocyte sedimentation rate (ESR), full blood count, renal function tests, blood glucose, liver function tests, bone profile, creatinine kinase, thyroid function tests and a chest X-ray. The blood test results returned after 2 days and showed a raised ESR of 70 mm/hour with all the other tests normal.

The GP informs the patient 'I am happy to have found the cause for your muscle pains which will improve dramatically with steroid tablets'. He prescribes 20 mg of oral prednisolone daily. However, at the next review the patient admits only minimal improvement. The GP doubles the dose of steroids. Just before the patient leaves the consulting room the receptionist comes in with the result of the chest X-ray. It reports 'Shadowing left upper hilar area. Possibly infective or neoplastic cause. Suggest repeat chest X-ray after 2 weeks.'

Questions

- What condition was the GP treating initially?
- What is differential diagnosis following the chest X-ray result?
- What tests would you arrange?
- Do you need to change any treatment?
- What do you tell the patient?

The GP initially treated the patient for polymyalgia rheumatica as the patient presented with the typical symptoms of this condition. The failure to respond to steroid therapy puts the accuracy of the diagnosis into doubt.

!

Following the chest X-ray result the differential diagnosis includes lung cancer, pneumonia and tuberculosis.

Lung cancer can cause proximal muscle weakness and would explain the slow progression of symptoms over a year. The patient might well suffer with an additional pneumonia caused by airway obstruction from the lung cancer. Given the age of the patient a hilar shadow might represent an old tuberculosis infection that has become active again. The GP will be worried that he might have accelerated the infection through the steroid treatment he has prescribed. The GP must order a repeat chest X-ray, requesting that the results be faxed to the surgery urgently: the result might trigger a referral, under the 2-week rule, to the chest clinic. The GP will also order three consecutive early-morning sputum samples to check cytology for lung cancer, and sputum culture for the acid fast bacilli of tuberculosis.

The steroid treatment has not resulted in any improvement of patient symptoms and should be stopped. It should be safe to stop it immediately, rather than in a graduated fashion, as the patient has no past history of adrenal suppression and has been on treatment for only a short time. The patient should be started on a suitable antibiotic to treat a possible pneumonia.

The GP will be caught off guard having had little time to prepare himself to deal with the new findings. One way of informing the patient of the suspected lung cancer would be to review the findings and progress so far with the patient. Summarising the initial presentation and blood test findings, reviewing the suspected diagnosis and failure to respond to the steroid treatment creates the context to allow the GP to add in the chest X-ray findings. At this moment in time it is not clear if the patient has lung cancer, but the suspicion is high. The way the GP handles giving the news to the patient will vary with how much the patient already suspects a malignant diagnosis and so it is very important to check the patient's ideas and concerns. If he does suspect cancer, one can help him to maintain hope by sharing with him the differential diagnoses. The doctor will need to use his professional judgment about how much information to divulge to an unaware patient. However, if the suspicion is firm enough to justify a 2-week referral, the patient must be informed of the possible malignant cause.

⚷ KEY POINTS

- It is important to take a full history at the initial assessment and follow up all abnormal findings.
- Doctors need to reassess the working diagnosis when a patient fails to respond to treatment.
- Breaking bad news is a process that primarily depends on your patient's prior knowledge, understanding and suspicion about their symptoms.

CASE 38: FERTILITY PROBLEM

History

A 26-year-old woman presents with a problem of irregular periods. Since coming off the combined oral contraceptive pill 9 months ago she has menstruated only twice, her last menstruation being 3 months ago. She is in a stable relationship and she and her partner have had regular sexual intercourse hoping that she would conceive after coming off the pill. She did a pregnancy test 2 days previously and it was negative. Before she started on the contraceptive pill she used to have irregular periods with cycles between 28 days and 3 months. She does complain of mild acne and some facial hair. She has no significant past medical history, in particular no past history of abdominal operations or pelvic inflammatory disease, and has never been pregnant. Her partner has no children. Neither of the couple smoke, they are not on any medications and they drink a little alcohol socially, and only occasionally. She works as an office administrator and her partner is a travel agent. Her maternal grandmother suffers with late-onset diabetes mellitus.

Examination

Her records show a body mass index of 26.3 and a blood pressure of 126/74 mmHg.

INVESTIGATIONS

Previously a doctor had ordered blood tests and a pelvic ultrasound with the following results.

	Patient result	Follicular phase	Mid-cycle peak	Luteal phase
FSH	5.8 IU/L	4–12 IU/L	6–25 IU/L	2–10 IU/L
LH	19.7 IU/L	1–18 IU/L	20–90 IU/L	1–19 IU/L

(FSH, follicle-stimulating hormone; LH, luteinizing hormone)

Pelvic ultrasound: The uterus is retroverted and measures $4.6 \times 3.8 \times 4.5$ cm. The endome-trial lining has a smooth uniform echo texture and is 9 mm thick. The right ovary has a volume of 14.5 mL and contains multiple cysts, more than 25, most of which are located within the periphery of the ovary. The left ovary has a total of 16 cysts and a volume of just 12 mL.

Questions

- What is the patient's diagnosis?
- Which tests are needed to investigate her infertility?
- How would you follow up your patient long term?

ANSWER

The patient suffers from polycystic ovary syndrome (PCOS). The raised LH and a LH: FSH ratio approaching 3 are indicative of this condition. The ultrasound findings of the right ovary reach the diagnostic criteria. Your patient has been tested thoroughly already. However 30 per cent of couples that have a fertility problem have a multifactorial cause for this. The next step would be to do a sperm count of her partner. If the sperm count is normal and they fail to conceive with first line treatment, tubal patency testing would be the next investigation. Many women with PCOS have insulin resistance. Patients with this condition have an increased risk of developing diabetes, high blood pressure, and a high cholesterol later in life. Some doctors advocate annual blood pressure, blood glucose and lipid checks. Amenorrhoea owing to PCOS is a risk factor in developing uterine cancer in later life. Further management includes rubella testing and starting her on folic acid in case she falls pregnant, as well as minimizing alcohol intake, reducing weight and doing a sensible amount of exercise if she is not already doing this. Weight reduction and increasing exercise levels appear to reduce the risk of associated disease as well as increase fertility.

 KEY POINTS

- Problems with fertility can be extremely distressing for patients and their partners and require a sensible and supportive response from GPs.
- Lifestyle changes can be more efficacious than pharmacological therapy for many diseases.

History

It is your turn on night duty at the local deputizing service. You have been very busy in the last few weeks, because of a national outbreak of influenza. You get a call from the wife of one of your own practice's patients, the headmaster of a local school. She apologizes for disturbing you, and thinks her husband has flu: she is merely seeking telephone advice. She says he has been feverish for 2–3 days with aches and pains, and is now sweating and shivering. He also has a slight rash on his hands. The general symptoms are entirely typical of the cases of influenza you have been seeing lately, and which normal respond to the usual regime of fluids and paracetamol. However, the rash does not quite fit the story. You decide to visit the patient.

Examination

The patient is a 45-year-old man, in bed, looking flushed and sweaty, and very apologetic for troubling you. His temperature is 39°C, his pulse 98 beats/minute and his chest is clear. He does have a scattered punctate reddish-brown rash on the palms of his hands, and a few similar spots on his forearms, but nowhere else.

Questions

- Is this patient seriously ill?
- What further clinical features could you look for?
- What immediate treatment is advised?
- Is there any advice to give to his family?

Using your pocket lens as a glass, you find the spots do not blanch on pressure. It is just possible he has meningococcal infection, but there is no neck stiffness. However, you decide to give him an intramuscular injection of benzylpenicillin, 1.2 G, in the upper outer quadrant of his buttock. You also arrange immediate admission to hospital, warning ambulance control that you suspect the case may be infectious. The following morning you phone the local consultant in Communicable Disease Control, to notify her of your suspected diagnosis, and complete and send the Infectious Diseases Notification form. You ask the consultant for advice on prophylaxis of the family (oral rifampicin or similar, possibly with meningitis A, C or other immunization depending on laboratory results), the school (no routine precautions unless there are more cases) and yourself (no prophylaxis needed).

Later that day you visit the hospital to find your patient in the intensive care unit, intubated and infused, with a diagnosis of *Neisseria meningitidis* group C confirmed. His wife by his side confirms that she and her two teenage children have been given prophylaxis. A month later the patient appears in your surgery, fully recovered and with no neurological or cognitive damage. He is only aware of his narrow escape by the increased solicitude of his family. You offer him a further fortnight off work, to convalesce, and he finally returns to teaching, fully fit, 6 weeks after the onset of his illness.

 KEY POINTS

- Just because 'there's a lot of it about', do not assume that the next case is the same as the previous half-dozen. Be aware of red-flag signs or symptoms, and cultivate your 'sixth sense' of something not quite right about a case.
- Check your emergency supplies in your bag, immediately replacing any you use, and ensuring they are all in date. Most of the time the drugs have to be discarded unused, a necessary expense for a GP.
- Refresh your knowledge of current advice on treatment and prophylaxis of infections, using the *British National Formulary* and the website of the Health Protection Agency.
- Offer support to the family of a patient with serious disease: they may have questions that they are too shy to ask at the hospital.

History

A single 32-year-old Kenyan-born secretary attends your emergency surgery. She reports that the day before yesterday she developed some flu-like symptoms with a headache and muscle pains. She lost her appetite, did not eat dinner and went to bed hoping to sleep it off. Yesterday she stayed at home and later that day she suddenly developed severe coldness and shivering (rigors) followed by drenching sweats, vomiting and flushing. Once the vomiting settled she took some paracetamol and felt a bit better. In the night she had another of these episodes and so decided to see the doctor.

Further questioning reveals she travelled to Kenya 8 weeks previously to attend the christening of her sister's child. Your computer records show that she saw the nurse before her journey and was prescribed mefloquine tablets (one tablet weekly to be started 2 weeks before travel until 4 weeks after return). She admits to taking the first two tablets only as they made her feel funny. She read the leaflet and became concerned that the tablets might cause her to become 'mad' and then she forgot to take the tablets with her on the journey. She was also worried about taking the tablets because she was hoping to have another child soon. In Kenya nobody took tablets and her family does not use mosquito nets. She thought that if her family was fine, and nobody was using mosquito nets, perhaps the risk for malaria was not so high. Returning from holiday she felt well and 2 weeks later she binned the remaining tablets.

Examination

On examination the patient looks unwell. Her sclera are jaundiced and she has cervical lymphadenopathy. Her temperature is 39.4°C, resting heart rate 104 beats/minute, blood pressure 123/87 mmHg and respiratory rate 18 breaths/minute. Her liver is palpable below the costal edge and tender. The GP is not certain if he can feel the tip of her spleen.

Questions
- What is your diagnosis?
- How should the GP manage this patient?

ANSWER

The patient has all the clinical symptoms suggestive of acute falciparum malaria that, in its most severe form, cerebral malaria, has a high mortality rate. The diagnosis is confirmed by blood microscopy (thick film). In partially treated patients bone marrow smears are an alternative.

About 2000 patients return to the UK from travel abroad with malaria each year and patients should be strongly encouraged to take chemoprophylaxis. In this case, the patient was reassured by her family's seeming lack of perception of danger. While malaria is a common illness in Africa conveying a relative immunity to those that have had previous infections, our patient is unlikely having maintained this immunity while living in the UK. For patients born and brought up in malarial areas immunity develops slowly and is rapidly lost if the person moves away.

Patients with acute and severe malaria need intense monitoring and observation. A full blood count might show anaemia, raised white cell count and often thrombocytopenia. Patients are at risk of hypoglycaemia and the liver function tests might reveal liver involvement. Urine analysis can show haematuria (black-water fever). Treatment needs the supervision of a specialist, preferably in cooperation with a microbiologist or tropical disease specialist.

 KEY POINTS

- Always include a travel history when patients present with non-specific symptoms.
- A traveller returning from a malarial area and presenting with flu-like symptoms has malaria until the disease has been ruled out.
- It is important to check compliance with medication.
- Patients born and raised in malarial areas may have a false sense of security when they return home.
- This is malaria but also have a high index of suspicion for early *Human immunodeficiency virus* (HIV) infection for anybody with a fever, rash and sore throat.

CASE 41: FOOT DROP

History

A 22-year-old college student attends the evening emergency clinic and walks in on crutches. He was injured during a college football match in Germany 1 week ago as a result of a two-foot tackle from a player on the German team. At first he was able to get up and limp and he continued to play football for another 10 minutes when, because of the pain, he was replaced. With rest his pain settled; his team won and they had a big party that night. The next day he was suffering more pain but his coach dismissed his pain as cramps. Later that night he was admitted to hospital. The doctor injected some dye into his foot and X-rayed his leg. The student was told he had a deep vein thrombosis (DVT) and was started on injections to thin his blood. Three days later he was discharged on crutches and given syringes containing the blood-thinning medication. The student had managed his first days well on crutches. However, yesterday he had fallen several times on the stairs of his parent's house and today while walking on crutches he had fallen unprovoked.

Examination

The GP finds good foot pulses and a bruise over the outside of the ankle with tenderness stressing the lateral ligaments. There is deep tenderness over the outer upper aspect of the shin and the anterior muscles, and the student reports worsening of the pain in this area on walking. No losses in sensation are found, but the student remembers severe pins and needles over the area of tenderness initially. There is weakness when trying to pull the foot upwards against resistance and pain when the foot and toes are bent downwards.

Questions
- What is the diagnosis?
- Is contrast venography the appropriate investigation?
- How would you manage this patient?
- What is the prognosis for the student?

ANSWER

The student is suffering from subacute anterior compartment syndrome. This condition is characterized by the six 'Ps': 'pain', 'pallor', 'paraesthesia', 'pulselessness', 'paralysis' and 'pressure' on passive extension of the compartment. Our student reported pain early. Characteristically the pain is deep and constant, is poorly localized, seems out of proportion to the severity of the injury, and can be aggravated by passive stretching of the muscle group involved. Paraesthesia of the affected cutaneous nerves is another typical sign. The pulse can be found as long the arterial pressure is higher than the pressure causing the compartment syndrome. Paralysis sets in later: in this patient it took a week to develop.

> Acute anterior compartment syndrome is caused by trauma of a limb causing bleeding and swelling inside the muscle compartment and is a surgical emergency. Chronic compartment syndrome is caused by over-usage of a muscle group causing the muscle to over-develop and put pressure on the surrounding sheath and can be seen in athletes.

The admitting doctor suspected a DVT. Contrast venography has been considered the gold standard in diagnosing the condition, but has been superseded by Doppler ultrasound, which has become the standard imaging procedure. It is of no surprise that the venogram showed a positive finding as the pressure rise in the muscle compartment diminishes venous return. The admitting doctor made a common diagnostic error by closing the diagnostic enquiry too early. The history and clinical signs and symptoms of the football injury did not fit the diagnosis of a DVT: the pain was too severe for the underlying injury and patients with venous symptoms do not develop paraesthesia or paralysis. The positive imaging result seemed to confirm the misdiagnosis and the doctor initiated the wrong treatment: anticoagulation might actually have worsened the condition.

The student should be told to rest the leg, elevate it and cool it with ice to reduce the swelling, and be given a non-steroidal analgesic to reduce the pain. As the pain is already greatly reduced since the time of admission, surgical treatment is probably unnecessary. However, it would be wise to phone an orthopaedic consultant to discuss the management. The anticoagulation treatment should be stopped. The majority of patients with subacute and chronic compartment syndrome regain normal muscle function after paralysis. After the initial rest period they need to be encouraged to do muscle strengthening exercises. Patients with acute compartment syndrome might lose function permanently if urgent surgical treatment is delayed.

 KEY POINTS

- Closing a diagnostic enquiry early by ignoring certain signs and symptoms may lead to misdiagnosis. In the case above the initiated test falsely confirmed the misdiagnosis.
- A positive test result might have other causes than the expected.
- If you are faced with additional signs that do not fit the working diagnosis, restart your diagnostic enquiry.

CASE 42: GENETIC DISORDER

History

The GP has been seeing a 63-year-old woman with a recent suicide attempt, an alcohol problem, hypertension and a family history of Huntington's disease. This scenario is further explained in Case 76. The woman lives alone and has a brother with Huntington's about whom she is very anxious. The GP is concerned that the patient gets proper support to deal with her problems and anxieties. The GP arranges to see the patient regularly. They explore her physical, psychological and social situation, focusing on her hypertension, low mood and suicide risk, alcohol problem and the possibility of her having Huntington's disease. As part of these sessions the GP and the patient spend some time talking about whether genetic testing might be appropriate at this stage. The patient has cared for her mother and seen her brother suffering from Huntington's disease: her mother died from pneumonia, one of the sequelae of Huntington's, after a long and debilitating illness and her brother is now wheelchair bound, confused and unable to care for himself. She has also experienced and seen the effect that such a genetic disorder has on families: her brother has three children in their 20s who live with the possibility that they may have the disorder. None have yet been tested. The patient, up until this point, has decided that she would rather not know whether or not she has the gene. She has reasoned that it would not make a difference to the way she lives her life whether or not she knows. However, recently, she has been more anxious about the future and about who would care for her were she to develop the symptoms of the disease. This was a big part of the reason she had been feeling low and starting to drink more heavily. She is worried that her symptoms of low mood and anxiety may be early signs of Huntington's disease – or are they normal given her situation?

As part of their discussions the GP explains the services available to diagnose and care for her were she to have the disease. They also talk about the progression of the disease and how it is usually a slow deterioration with potentially many initial good years of life. The patient decides to be tested for the Huntington's gene. Unfortunately, the test result reveals that she does indeed have the disordered gene.

Questions
- What services are there available for dealing with a genetic disorder?
- How might the GP deal with the patient's alcohol problem and low mood?

ANSWER

Every patient should have access to a genetics clinic where counselling, diagnosis and long-term support can be provided. This service is also there to support the professionals that care for patients with genetic disorders, have a family history of a genetic disorder or who are at risk of genetic disease. Hereditary diseases are often rare and affected families require specialist advice and services. General practitioners are able to refer to such clinics. In this particular situation the regional genetics clinic has a special Huntington's Disease Clinic and the GP refers his patient to them. The clinic has also cared for her mother and is caring for her brother so they are aware of the family situation. This comforts the patient. Where a genetic disease is diagnosed there are usually special organizations that support people affected by the disorder as well as providing information and advice to family, friends and health-care professionals. In the UK there is a Huntington's Disease Association, which is a charitable organization. The patient is put in touch with them and they visit her at home and invite her to their regular meetings. The patient finds them of great support. They also send the GP information about their service and make themselves available to support the GP in this patient's care should this be needed.

There are usually a number of services available for the care of patients with alcohol problems and low mood. Generally, the mental health services do not directly deal with patients with alcohol problems until these have been resolved, although some regions have dual clinics. In the case of this patient the GP gives her a number of options for alcohol counselling and she chooses the service that comes to the surgery for consultations. This proves successful. She has not had a drink since her suicide attempt and the weekly sessions assist her in considering preventive measures so that her drinking does not become a problem again. The GP also considers her low mood. In this situation the GP does not refer her to the mental health service, counsellors in the community or the practice counsellor but rather counsels her herself. She is put on antidepressants (a selective serotonin reuptake inhibitor, or SSRI, in view of the danger of overdose). There is a concern that this symptom may be an early sign of Huntington's disease. Over the next few months things settle down for the patient and a good patient–doctor relationship means that ongoing care and support is possible.

 KEY POINTS

- Genetic diseases such as this are uncommon in general practice. However, when they do occur the patient requires expert care and attention.
- Take time and a number of consultations to work through the situation so that the patient is not overwhelmed any more than they are already.
- Think of the whole person and address physical, psychological, social and spiritual concerns.

CASE 43: GIFTS

History

A 56-year-old business executive attends his GP for a review appointment for his lower back pain. Ten days previously he had needed an emergency visit. He had been working in his garden and while twisting, lifting tree branches, he had experienced the sudden onset of severe lower back pain. He had collapsed to the ground but had managed to get back into the house by crawling. He had taken pain-killers and rested overnight, but on the day of the visit he had felt even worse. The GP had taken a history and examined the patient and diagnosed simple lower back pain. He had reassured the patient, given an non-steroidal anti-inflammatory drug (NSAID) injection, and prescribed more analgesia which had been delivered by the chemist the same day. Now the patient reports that he is 99 per cent back to normal because of the 'marvellous treatment' that he received. He reminds the GP of the difficulties that he had experienced finding his property, necessitating three phone calls on route asking for directions: 'You need some technical help finding your patients, doctor'. The patient asks to have a repeat of his prescription items: 'The shampoo and cream that you provided me with has cleared my skin perfectly and my hay fever is so much better controlled this year'. Looking back at the records the GP sees that he had diagnosed the patient with seborrhoeic dermatitis on a new patient check 2 months ago. He had prescribed antifungal creams and shampoo and the patient's condition had responded well. He remembered that the patient, at that time, had given him an expensive aftershave as a sign of appreciation. On another occasion the GP had explained how to take the nasal steroid drops that were given to treat the patient's hay fever. He made a schematic drawing explaining the process. The patient was surprised that he had not known how to take his long-standing treatment and was quite taken with the drawing, requesting the GP to sign it: 'You might become a famous artist in the future'. Later, the patient had sent him aquarelle paper with coloured pastels. The GP had felt uncomfortable accepting this generous gift, but his fellow doctors told him that he had earned it. Three days later the GP receives a parcel from his patient containing a state-of-the-art satellite navigation system with a note from the patient: 'Now you won't get lost in the country anymore'.

Questions
- Which guidance governs the rules for doctors accepting gifts from patients?
- Why do patients offer gifts to doctors?
- Why might this GP feel uncomfortable accepting this gift?

ANSWER

The General Medical Council, in its document 'Good Medical Practice', provides clear guidance to doctors about receiving gifts: 'You must be honest and open in any financial arrangements with patients. In particular, you ... must not encourage patients to give, lend or bequeath money or gifts that will directly or indirectly benefit you. You must not ask for or accept any inducement gift or hospitality which may affect the way you prescribe for, treat or refer patients'. Many trusts have procedures for their staff, regulating gifts from patients by setting an acceptable upper value for gifts received and the way that gifts how must be declared. Cash gifts are usually not acceptable and GPs are contractually obliged to keep a register for gifts exceeding a value of £100.

Making a gift is a common socially acceptable way to show gratitude and appreciation. Most doctors are given between one and five gifts per year and the most common items are chocolate and alcoholic beverages or other food items. This patient gave thoughtful, fitting and humorous gifts. However, in this situation, the doctor and patient have not known each other long and it is worrying that the value of gifts seems to increase with each item. The patient might perceive a friendship or may want to build a friendly relationship. His last gift might be perceived as patronizing as most GPs have very good local knowledge of the practice area. On the other hand, the GP might be afraid that rejecting this generous gift might upset his patient endangering the development of a good patient–doctor relationship.

Doctors appreciate 'thank you cards' and small gifts. The cards can be used to provide evidence of good relationships with patients in annual appraisals. Larger gifts can feel less comfortable. The doctor might fear that the patient is trying to build up an obligation allowing them in future to ask for special treatment in terms of access to services and prescriptions. Generous gifts or legacies might upset the donor's family provoking complaints to the General Medical Council.

Sometimes doctors feel that they have not deserved a gift. This is especially true if they perceive that they have not provided the best normal services to the patient. Most doctors judge whether it is right to accept a gift by the following rule: if the local newspaper published the transaction would they feel ashamed or would their patients be upset? Many surgeries have a league of friends that raises funds for their surgery. The money raised is commonly used for buying additional medical equipment or improving areas for patient use, for example buying toys or providing a TV for the waiting room.

 KEY POINTS

- Gifts from patients are common and a socially acceptable way of showing appreciation for the doctor's good work.
- Doctors should be mindful when they accept generous gifts from patients.

CASE 44: GYNAECOMASTIA

History

Your next patient is a heavily built 12-year-old boy, attending the local comprehensive school, with a typical interest in football. His mother has brought him because they have noticed a lump in his chest, which has been present for a few weeks. It is causing him no pain, but bothers her because she herself had breast cancer, successfully treated a few years ago.

Examination

You find a smooth, firm, round mass just under his right nipple, about 2 cm in diameter, which is not tender. The left side is normal. He is slightly overweight, with a body mass index of 26 measured on a growth chart for boys from 2–20 years of age that the GP downloads from the North American National Center for Health Statistics website.

Questions

- What can you tell the boy and his mother about this condition?
- What alternatives should you consider?
- What opportunistic health-care issues arise in this case?

ANSWER

At this age, the physiological changes of puberty are by far the most likely explanation. Over the next year or so, the swelling should subside, though it is quite likely also to affect the other side. It does not generally indicate abnormal hormones. As a precaution, you ask to review him in 3–6 months' time if it has not improved. You can reassure him that he is not changing sex, and his mother that he does not have cancer. True gynaecomastia is a persistent, usually bilateral, enlargement of breast tissue in males. In this case, a quick trawl through his records shows that he has had his MMR (measles, mumps, and rubella) immunizations, and has not had mumps. A simple examination of his genitalia show normal testes and penis, excluding rarities such as Klinefelter's syndrome. He not in the age-range to expect liver disease, anti-androgen or digoxin therapy. Most cases of persistent gynaecomastia are idiopathic, though there have been some studies suggesting that environmental oestrogens (metabolites of the oral contraceptive pill, contaminating water supplies through ineffective sewage treatment) may be contributing to an increase in incidence. Obesity can give an impression of breast enlargement in men and boys. You can discuss his diet, and use his interest in football to enhance his exercise regime.

KEY POINTS

- Do not dismiss a patient's concern over a minor problem as trivial: it is obviously not trivial for them, or they would not be consulting you.
- Treat the patient with respect, demonstrate that you understand their worry and follow up the case even if you expect natural recovery.
- The perception of body-image changes markedly during puberty. The sense of what is normal has to accommodate the physiological alteration to anatomy and emotion; it is common knowledge that this is a troublesome period for boys and girls alike, and their parents.
- If the problem does not resolve as expected, be prepared to reconsider your diagnosis.

CASE 45: HEADACHE

History

It has been a busy year. You have joined a new practice, gained a new baby, taken on an honorary Trustee post with a charity, and now have to fit in tutorials for the medical students – all on top of the daily routine of surgeries, reports, home visits and out-of-hours sessions – and now you are getting one of your migraine headaches again. You have been getting these increasingly frequently of late, now almost weekly. The headaches usually occur on a Friday night and can last through the weekend – exhausting when this is the time for relaxation after a busy week. However, they can come at any time and when they happen at work life gets very difficult. The frontal pain is devastating, you are cold and sweaty and you have to dash to the toilet between patients to be sick. If you could only go home, lie down in a darkened room, and sleep for an hour you know you will feel completely well again. Instead, you take a couple of soluble aspirins in water, which does relieve the pain considerably.

Questions

- What are the benefits and disadvantages of self-medication in this case?
- Whom can you ask for advice?

ANSWER

Many people with migraine recognize that it is a self-limiting, if recurrent, problem. Simple analgesics are sometimes effective, but the side-effects of aspirin limit its usefulness. More specific remedies are combinations with metoclopramide, or a 5-HT1 (serotonin receptor) antagonist such as sumatriptan. When you subsequently find yourself woken at night with severe indigestion, you are forced to register with a GP to seek help. The consequent endoscopy reveals a self-inflicted aspirin-induced gastric ulcer. A short course of lansoprazole cures that. Your GP also recommends a beta-blocker to control your coincidental hypertension, which has the double merit of abolishing the migraine and allowing you to get life insurance for a mortgage.

The General Medical Council in their 2006 booklet, *Good Practice in Prescribing Medicines*, advises that 'doctors should, wherever possible, avoid treating themselves or anyone with whom they have a close personal relationship, and should be registered with a GP outside their family. Controlled drugs can present particular problems, occasionally resulting in a loss of objectivity leading to drug misuse and misconduct'.

 KEY POINTS

- Don't say 'yes' to every demand made on you. You have to learn to pace your life: a sick doctor is useless to patients, and as a human being you are entitled to the same consideration as you would give your own patients.
- If you are unfortunately unwell, seek advice from a trusted GP, who can view your problem dispassionately, and guide you through the maze of the NHS if needed.
- You will avoid incurring the wrath of the General Medical Council if you do not prescribe for yourself.

History

The GP is visited by a man who is seen infrequently at the practice. He explains that he is about to be made homeless and asks for help. He is 23 years old and is at present living with his girlfriend. He has had a difficult life. He was adopted at birth and was one of three children; the other two were not adopted. His upbringing was not easy as he never got on with his adoptive father who was very hard on him compared with his siblings. His physical health was fine apart from the usual childhood illnesses. He struggled at school, particularly in interactions with his peers and with cognitive functioning. When he was 8 years old educational psychologists were involved and he was given the diagnosis of dyslexia. There were no special schools near to where they were living at that time and so he was given extra lessons and support but always found schooling difficult. From the age of 12 years old he was often truant from school. He was prone to rages and his peers were very wary of interacting with him. Educational psychologists were once again involved and he and his parents attended the local child and adolescent mental health service for some sessions. His behaviour improved somewhat and he stayed on at his school until GCSEs when he passed four papers. He then left school and worked in a video shop for a few months, leaving after an argument with the manager; since then he has worked in a number of jobs. For the last 6 months he has been unemployed although he has had a few temporary jobs through the Job Centre. He has been with his present girlfriend for 1 year but recently she has asked him to leave as she is tired of his irritability and inability to hold down a job. She has told him that she would like him out of the house by the end of the month. He has no money set aside and not enough money coming in to rent a flat. His family is unable to help him financially to get housing and he does not want to return home as he does not get on well with his father. He tells the GP that his father thinks he is 'a loser'.

Questions
- What would the GP focus on in the consultation?
- What services would be able to help this young man?

ANSWER

The GP will need to get him back for a further consultation as this introduction to the problem has already taken 15 minutes. She arranges for the patient to have a double appointment at the end of the surgery 3 days later. There are a number of areas that the GP wishes to explore with the patient to do with his physical, psychological and social health. The GP finds out that the young man has been physically well but does binge drink once and sometimes twice a week when he drinks about six pints of beer with his friends, smokes about 20 cigarettes daily and occasionally smokes cannabis and uses cocaine. He does want to stop binge drinking, he drinks little the rest of the week and his weekly intake is about 15 units. The patient talks about not believing in himself and worrying that he will never be good enough to live a normal, healthy life. The GP diagnoses him as having moderately severe depression (with a score of 17 out of 27 on the patient health questionnaire, PHQ-9; see Table in Case 62). He is not suicidal and has never wanted to 'end it all'. He tells the GP that he can sometimes fly into rages and frightens his girlfriend although he has never physically hurt her. He is very sad that his girlfriend wants to end their relationship as he is very fond of her. He hopes that if can sort himself out and find a job they can get back together.

The doctor has elucidated a number of problems: a low level of confidence and self-esteem, cigarette smoking, a non-dependent alcohol and drug problem, depression, a problem with anger, and an inability to find and hold down a job.

There are a number of services that could help this man. It is suggested that he goes to the local housing service for help with his housing problem and the GP writes a letter pointing out that he is vulnerable and in need of urgent housing. He is also referred to the community drug and alcohol service where he can receive counselling and get help with anger management. The patient does not feel that he is ready to stop smoking but is keen to do so if the other problems can be sorted out. Finally, an appointment is made with an employment advisor who works in the neighbourhood with the idea of helping him access suitable training. The patient expresses an interest in being a car mechanic and the GP hopes that the advisor can assist him in working towards this goal. Another appointment is made to see him in a week to talk about progress.

 KEY POINTS

- Young men tend to turn to health services only when they are desperate.
- Young homeless men are extremely vulnerable: they are more at risk from accidents, mental health problems, suicide, alcohol- and drug-related illness, liver disease and respiratory infections.
- Find out about services available for young men who are in difficulty and try hard to keep them engaged.

History

A 72-year-old woman comes to see her GP after seeing the practice nurse for a new patient check. The nurse had arranged blood tests and to the patient's surprise she had received a letter from the practice asking her to see the doctor because of a high cholesterol with normal triglycerides. Together with the patient the GP puts her data into a computer-based coronary heart disease (CHD) and stroke risk calculator: no evidence of existing arteriosclerotic disease, 72 years of age, female, systolic blood pressure 142 mmHg, diastolic blood pressure 86 mmHg, smoker, total cholesterol 6.8 mmol/L, high-density lipoprotein (HDL) cholesterol 1.0 mmol/L, not diabetic and no evidence of left ventricular hypertrophy. The calculation for the risk of a primary disease event in the next 10 years is 24 per cent for CHD and 8.1 per cent for stroke. The first number is displayed in red indicating a raised value.

The patient is concerned as she feels well. The GP explains that the calculator gives a prediction of the likelihood of heart attack and stroke over the next 10 years in women of her age and health status. 'Of 100 women of your age with a similar blood pressure, cholesterol and smoking status, 24 will have a heart attack in the next 10 years. Let's look what your risk would be if you were 40 years younger'. He changes her age to 32 years and the calculated CHD risk drops to 2.2 per cent. The GP explains that he cannot make her younger but that there are some factors in the calculation that they can change, such as lowering her blood pressure and cholesterol and stopping smoking. He changes the systolic blood pressure to 128 mmHg and the risk drops to 21.6 per cent, but the number remains red. Next, he changes the total cholesterol to 5.0 mmol/L and the risk reduces further to 15.8 per cent. 'See, by lowering your blood pressure and cholesterol your risk reduces by more than one-third. However, the red number shows that you continue to live with a higher than desirable level of risk for heart attack and stroke. Let's see what would happen if you stopped smoking'. The risk calculation for a non-smoker comes down to 10 per cent and the number is now in green. 'Look, stopping smoking would bring your risk down to an acceptable range' states the doctor. 'I did not know how much of a difference smoking makes' exclaims the patient. 'What do I need to do now, doctor, to keep healthy?'

Questions

- What are the dangers of informing patients of their risk factors?
- Is the doctor right confirming the patient's belief she is healthy?

ANSWER

It is important to distinguish between an actual disease and the risk factor for that disease. A raised cholesterol or a high blood pressure are not diseases in themselves, but they do increase the risk of disease, namely atherosclerotic disease affecting different organs. This patient feels well and has no manifestations of atherosclerotic disease. Even with a risk of nearly one in four of having a heart attack in the next 10 years, she is more likely to develop coronary artery disease without suffering a heart attack. Patients, health professionals and the media often blur this important distinction. We hear of epidemics of risk factors as if they were contagious. It seems as if risk factors have become the 'new' diseases. In an occupational health study a sample of normotensive factory workers at a routine medical check-up were told that they suffered from high blood pressure. At the next medical they were informed that the diagnosis of hypertension was not true. Follow-up showed that the group of workers who were falsely informed of a raised blood pressure had a significantly increased number of days off work owing to ill health compared with their controls. In medical practice we see many patients who tell us that they 'suffer' from high cholesterol or high blood pressure associating many symptoms with these risk factors. It can be frustrating for doctors trying to contradict patients' strongly held misconceptions.

Patients' health is a precious asset. The population spends a fortune each year buying food and vitamin supplements in order to maintain good health. Patients' feelings of health are not solely related to the absence of disease and their belief in their good health can be easily shaken. More important than the real risk of the disease is the perceived risk of being vulnerable to a disease event. This feeling of vulnerability becomes even more important when the risk in question is (or felt to be) outside the patients' control. For example the risk of becoming ill through 'mad cow disease' is remote, but when it first became news it caused a lot of fear and was kept in the headlines for a long time. The risk of dying in road traffic is real, but it provokes less fear and attention. Doctors should maintain health and allow patients to take charge of risk factors. Starting medication is often seen by patients as a sign of disease, making them reluctant to commit to treatment. Allowing patients to see medication as a gift that is helping them to stay healthy can overcome this problem.

 KEY POINTS

- It is important to maintain the distinction between disease and risk factors.
- Doctors should aim to maintain health and allow patients to take charge of risk factors.

History

You have been monitoring your patient's blood pressure for a number of years. The readings fluctuate between 115/70 mmHg and 160/95 mmHg, with a tendency to rise over the last 6 months or so. To begin with, he was on no medication, but about 2 years ago he started bendroflumethiazide, 5 mg daily, which has helped slightly and serves to keep his incipient ankle oedema at bay. He is a cheerful, local car mechanic, white, married, with four children. He is now 54 years old. He is a non-smoker, drinks a beer or two most nights, and is otherwise well with a body mass index (BMI) of 23. He has reached the point where you want to add a second hypotensive agent. He is a little doubtful, as he feels well, and does not want to risk any of the side-effects his friends have experienced, such as swollen ankles, tiredness and, most significantly, impotence.

INVESTIGATIONS	
A glance at his record shows the following recent test results.	
Fasting serum total cholesterol:	5.9 mmol/L
Ratio of total cholesterol to high-density lipoprotein:	3.8
Serum creatinine, estimated glomerular filtration rate (eGFR), electrolytes:	Normal
Fasting blood glucose:	3.5 mmol/L
Urinalysis:	Normal
Electrocardiogram :	Normal

Questions

- What are the possible consequences of inaction?
- What alternative or additional medication could you suggest?
- What side-effects might he expect?

ANSWER

You might want to run a 24-hour blood pressure monitoring if you suspect 'white-coat hypertension' as you do not want to add medication unless it is truly necessary. Strokes, heart attacks and renal failure are the serious sequelae of uncontrolled hypertension. Your computer calculates that his 10-year risk of a coronary heart disease or cerebrovascular event is 11 per cent. However, the charts are based on groups of people with untreated blood pressure and cholesterol so, although they can act as a guide, for those already receiving therapy it is safest to assume that the coronary heart disease (CHD) and stroke risk is higher than indicated.

Refer to the latest guidelines, for example in the *British National Formulary,* for the treatment of hypertension. For essential hypertension in a white patient who is younger than 55 years an angiotensin-converting enzyme (ACE) inhibitor is the current first line of treatment. Current thinking might also add a lipid-lowering statin and anti-thrombotic aspirin to the cocktail. For this patient, because he is already on a thiazide diuretic, the addition of an ACE inhibitor would be the next step. However, the patient is right: side-effects can occur and can be more of a problem to the patient than the asymptomatic disease: the full list of side-effects, published by the manufacturers, is disheartening. One thinks of gout, diabetes, hypokalaemia, hypotensive events, cold extremities, sleep disturbance, cough, renal impairment, swollen legs, and so on. Impotence can also occur with some of these agents. Even statins and aspirin can have untoward effects, such as muscle pains or dyspepsia. When starting a new treatment, you will need to mention at least the most common possible side-effects for him to look out for.

For a patient with an 'invisible' (i.e. asymptomatic) disease, you wish to offer an 'invisible' treatment (i.e. high blood pressure usually has no symptoms and the medicine should cause no effects noticeable to the patient, but the blood pressure is being lowered to great benefit, and hopefully with no side-effects). The results of the treatment are 'invisible' (the reduction in blood pressure can only be detected by someone measuring it), and the whole point of the exercise is that nothing should happen – no event such as a cerebrovascular accident (CVA) in the future. Furthermore, you cannot guarantee success, even with the best treatment; he could still have a heart attack or stroke, though his risks will be reduced on treatment. The whole premise is based on statistical studies of large populations.

At this point, it might be judicious to suggest that the patient goes away and thinks it over, perhaps pointing him to useful leaflets or internet sites, before he commits to a lifetime of medication. Increasing his exercise, relaxing, taking extra care with his diet and reducing salt intake may be an easier first step.

 KEY POINTS

- Keep up to date with treatment protocols.
- Provide the patient with information on efficacy and side-effects of medication.
- Take as much time as necessary; and it is prudent to come to management decisions together with the patient.

History

The GP is visited by a 35-year-old man who reports that he has been unable to sleep over the past few weeks. He has had a 2-month history of headaches and left eye pain. An initial check by the optometrist revealed nothing. He has recently been referred and seen by the ophthalmologists and they have diagnosed ocular myositis, an idiopathic inflammation of the extra-ocular muscles. They have prescribed prednisolone at an initial dose of 50 mg, as well as codeine phosphate 60 mg four times a day. His headaches and eye pain are better but he is still not well and the chronic pain has been very disabling. He has not been able to work as a builder for the last 4 months and is very concerned about his finances and his future. He lives with his girlfriend of 5 years in a rented flat. He has generally been a fit and healthy man and has seldom visited the general practice prior to this illness. He has had no serious illnesses and has not had a history of depression or psychosis. He is an ex-smoker and does drink a little too much alcohol at 20–30 units per week, mostly at the weekend. He has used cocaine and smoked cannabis occasionally in the past but does not now and does not use any other recreational drugs. He worked out at the gym before he got ill and wants to get back to his exercise but does not seem to have the motivation. He complains that his appetite has recently increased and that he has put on weight over the past few months. His mum and dad are still alive: his mum has osteoarthritis but is otherwise well at 60 years and his dad is 65 years old and has high blood pressure. Both his siblings are well and no-one in his family has had a major psychiatric illness.

On questioning him further the GP finds out that he has felt more irritable recently, with increased energy and racing thoughts. He also reports that he has times of feeling low, has lost interest in doing things and finds it hard to concentrate. His relationship with his girlfriend has been going downhill and he has taken to sleeping in the spare room so that he does not disturb her during the night. He tends to not to be able to go to sleep until about 2 a.m. and then wakes about 6 a.m. and cannot get back to sleep. He finds he is getting up and pacing around his room and not able to settle.

Examination

The GP notices that his speech seems pressured. General physical examination is normal apart from a body mass index of 27, having been 22 when he was well.

Questions
- What is the differential diagnosis?
- What options are possible for management?

ANSWERS

> The differential diagnosis includes bipolar disorder and substance-induced mood disorder.

Given that the symptoms have only started since the patient started on a high dose of prednisolone, that he is not taking recreational drugs and that he has no past history or any family history of psychosis or bipolar disorder the likely cause is the prednisolone.

The GP contacts the ophthalmologist and the psychiatrist. It is agreed to slowly reduce the prednisolone. The psychiatrists introduce olanzapine. However, the pain increases when the prednisolone is reduced below 15 mg daily and olanzapine is associated with drowsiness and depression. The prednisolone is slowly reduced over the next 2 months while azathioprine and cyclosporin are introduced for his ocular myositis with regular blood testing for liver and renal function as well as full blood counts. Calcium and vitamin D tablets are added to his medication regime while he is taking the steroids as he has been on over 7.5 mg of prednisolone for almost 6 months. Citalopram is added but he becomes manic again. Lithium is thus instituted and this has a better effect on the patient's mood swings. The ophthalmologists manage to stop the prednisolone without any increase in pain. The psychiatrist and the ophthalmologist see him regularly for monitoring. He is also seen by the practice employment counsellor and computer training is organized. He is given incapacity benefit.

 KEY POINTS

- Exact diagnosis is often not clear and symptoms can be multifactorial.
- Disease management is often a balance between the benefits of treatment and costs such as iatrogenic illness.
- In a situation such as this, close monitoring and a 'balancing act' is required, which is exhausting for the patient (and to a lesser extent for the doctor).

History

Your next patient is the 32-year-old mother of three children: a boy aged 8 years, a girl aged 5 years and a new baby boy aged 6 weeks. The eldest boy has learning and behaviour problems and has been labelled as moderately autistic. Her husband, originally from India, has had epilepsy for many years, although it is well controlled. She had a difficult pregnancy this time, with persistent vomiting requiring treatment with prochlorperazine, and the baby was born 4 weeks prematurely. However, he appears normal, is thriving, and is being successfully breast-fed. He has been brought for his routine 6-week development assessment. No problems are found, and his developmental age is consistent with his slight prematurity. His mother asks about immunization, and you describe the routine vaccines which are recommended. She is agreeable in principle, but has reservations about the MMR (measles, mumps, rubella) vaccine, as she has read newspaper articles and internet pages linking it with autism. She asks for the individual vaccines to be given separately, instead of in a combined vaccine.

Questions

- What routine immunizations are offered in the UK schedule for children?
- What explanation can you give her about the safety of the vaccines?
- What options can you offer her in this case?

ANSWER

The routine immunizations offered in the UK, as at January 2008, are:

- diphtheria/tetanus/pertussis (DTP)
- poliomyelitis (IPV)
- *Haemophilus influenzae* type b (Hib)
- pneumococcal infection (PCV)
- meningitis C (MenC)
- measles/mumps/rubella (MMR)

Non-routine immunizations that protect against tuberculosis (BCG – Bacille Calmette-Guérin) and hepatitis B (Hep B) are given to babies who are more likely to come into contact with these diseases than the general population. The exact immunization schedule does change so it is wise to keep up to date with Department of Health information and literature.

Protection against these diseases depends on a combination of group and individual immunity. Side-effects of all these vaccines are generally mild and self-limiting, and include fever (ameliorated with a dose of paracetamol or ibuprofen), and possible febrile convulsions (the parental history of epilepsy is not a contraindication to immunization here). Serious side-effects are very rare, though every surgery offering immunizations should have an anaphylaxis pack ready to hand 'just in case'. The risks should be balanced against the very real risks of contracting the diseases, and there is no doubt that the benefits far outweigh the risk of harm. In particular, the mother can be assured that repeated, extensive, carefully controlled studies have failed to show any link between the current vaccines and autism. Giving measles, mumps and rubella separately would increase the number of injections in the first years of life with no increase in safety. Furthermore, single-dose vaccines are not available via the NHS and she would need to consult a private doctor about this. You might ask her first to discuss this with her husband, and for both of them to consult with you. If she remains adamant, you will need to ask her to sign a form stating that she declines your advice, and accepts responsibility for the consequences to her child. This formality does tend to concentrate the mind on the serious nature of the decision. You would also wish to discuss her case with the health visitor, as this child is at risk of catching or transmitting infection in the Child Health Clinic.

In addition, this child should be offered (from birth onwards) a single dose of BCG vaccine, as his father was born in India, and relatives from the subcontinent may visit.

 KEY POINTS

- Just because the mother does not agree with your advice, this does not make her guilty of neglect.
- Parents are bombarded with advice from family, friends and the media, as well as from health professionals, and it is the parents' responsibility to decide what is best for their child.
- While explaining the possible consequences of her action you must respect her decision and continue to offer her medical advice and treatment as normal.

History

The patient in Case 34 returns to his GP for review 6 months after his radical prostate-ctomy. Being told that his life had been saved by the intervention had initially made him feel very positive and he had coped well in the immediate postoperative period. However, since the surgery he has been troubled by urinary incontinence. He was told that this was a common postoperative problem which usually improved within 6 weeks; the urology specialist nurse has shown him pelvic floor exercises but his incontinence has not improved. Two mid-stream urines have been negative for infection.

He has tried to return to work, but feels unable to do so. In his job as a landscape gar-dener, lifting heavy loads now causes him to be severely incontinent. He has tried to disguise his problem by wearing incontinence pads, but he has wet his pants on several occasions. He feels embarrassed and refuses to return to work until his incontinence problem is addressed. He has withdrawn from all social activities, starting to smoke again and leaving the house only to go to the corner shop to buy cigarettes. He now smokes 40 cigarettes a day.

On questioning he admits to problems getting to sleep and to early-morning waking and has been tearful on occasions. He has lost interest in his hobbies and has not attempted to have sexual intercourse with his wife. He feels very tired and has problems concentrating when watching the television or reading the newspaper. He has lost about half a stone since the operation despite the lack of physical exercise. He admits to suicidal thoughts, but denies any concrete plans. Asked to compare his emotional state to a previous epi-sode of depression he says that he feels much worse. He tells the GP that his family is very concerned about him and they had persuaded him to make the appointment.

When offered talking therapies or antidepressive medication he refuses both. He says that this depression is different to the previous episode. Last time the depression had occurred spontaneously, but this time all his problems are caused by his physical problems.

Questions
- How would you manage this patient?
- How would you follow him up?
- Is the patient at risk?

ANSWER

The patient is referred back to the consultant urologist for assessment and treatment of his persistent urinary incontinence. The urologist plans to operate by implanting an artificial sphincter device involving a magnetic valve. The doctor arranges to see the patient in a few days time. Patients in acute distress need to be monitored closely and this patient has many suicidal risk factors, including being male and having a long-standing illness. At review many patients show marked improvement if they have been listened to initially. The patient is acutely depressed and having suicidal thoughts. He has some serious risk factors of self-harm, but has a good social network to rely on. Close follow-up is important and specialist referral might be indicated if no improvement is detected or if the patient's condition deteriorates. Patients need explanations about depression. The patient assumed that depression has to have a spontaneous onset: patient ideas about illness can be erroneous or only partly right. A leaflet explaining depression would give the patient a chance to read about the illness and engage with treatment in his own time.

The patient fails to attend his follow-up appointment, being acutely admitted to hospital with a major anterior myocardial infarction. In the coronary care unit the patient suffers three cardiac arrests, but each time is successfully resuscitated. The echocardiogram on discharge shows impairment of ventricular function. The patient engages well with the cardiac rehabilitation and the rehabilitation team convinces him to stop smoking. Having had his life saved a second time, he develops a more philosophical view of life and his depression improves gradually as he gains physical strength. The myocardial infarction delayed the implantation of the artificial sphincter device only minimally and the device improves his urinary continence to a level that he is able to cope with.

He was at high risk of ischaemic heart disease being male, middle-aged and a heavy smoker. He has never had his cholesterol checked prior to the cardiac event and it proves to be mildly elevated. Depression and erectile dysfunction, his original symptom, are two disorders that are significantly associated with ischaemic heart disease. At present it is unclear if patients with these conditions should be screened for coronary artery disease or should qualify for primary prevention of ischaemic heart disease.

 KEY POINTS

- Apparently minor medical problems, such as urinary incontinence, can have a major impact on a patient's life.
- Seemingly unrelated medical conditions can, together, predispose a person to significant medical illnesses.

CASE 52: INSOMNIA

History

A 28-year-old man goes to see his GP with a 6-month history of insomnia. He is not known well at the practice, seldom going to the doctor. However, his wife has encouraged him to attend as he is becoming less able to cope with his work and more irritable around the house. He works in the city as an accountant in a large management firm. He tends to work late, arriving home about 8.30 p.m. He and his wife have dinner about 10 p.m. and he goes to bed at midnight. He has a problem falling asleep; sometimes wakes again about 4.30 a.m., and then later has to force himself to wake and get put of bed at 6.30 a.m. to prepare to go to work. His work has been more stressful recently with a lot of new projects and a takeover by an American company on the cards. He is not sure whether he will keep his job. His wife works as an editor of a magazine and works long hours. They live in a comfortable house that they own and have no children.

Although the patient is tired, irritable and at times anxious, he does not report having felt particularly 'down', depressed or hopeless over the past month, or having been bothered by having little interest or pleasure in doing things. The patient does not have any urinary problems or any pain and he has no medical history of note. He does not smoke but drinks too much alcohol at 28 units per week on average. He exercises three times a week at the gym and generally does this in the middle of the day, as well as cycling to work and back. His wife does not complain of him snoring and he does not wake during the night gasping or choking.

Examination

He has a normal blood pressure and is of normal weight. To make sure that depression is not a major contributor the GP administers the Patient Health Questionnaire (PHQ-9; see Table in Case 62). The patient reports trouble with sleep and tiredness nearly every day but does not report anything else on the questionnaire. His score is therefore 6 out of 27, which is defined as mild depression.

Questions
- Why does the GP explore these areas?
- What can be done to help?

ANSWER

The GP needs to ensure that there are no other reasons for his insomnia, for example depression, urinary problems, pain or sleep apnoea. The GP therefore takes a full history and does an examination.

The GP talks with him about his sleep hygiene. He does go to bed and gets up at the same time each day, although at the weekends he stays in bed a little longer. He does exercise most days. His bedroom is quiet and dark and at a comfortable temperature. He does not work in his bedroom and tends to relax in the hour before going to bed by watching TV or reading the newspaper. He does not drink caffeine before bed but does have two glasses of wine with his meal at 10 p.m. – he says this helps him sleep. He does not sleep or nap during the day. When he cannot get to sleep he tends to lie worrying about his work, trying to keep still so that he does not wake his wife sleeping soundly beside him.

The GP talks with him about a few simple measures that might help his sleep. He recommends that he tries to get back from work a little earlier and have an earlier evening meal. He also suggests that he does not drink wine at night as, although this might help the patient get to sleep, it can also cause him to wake up in the early morning. He also suggests that if he cannot sleep that he get up and participate in a quiet activity in another room until he feels sleepy again and that he should do this as many times in the night as needed. They talk about the fact that the last hour of TV or reading should be peaceful rather than exciting and that simple relaxation exercises, soothing music, a warm bath and a milky drink might help his sleep. They also talk about the anxiety related to his job and he agrees to see the practice counsellor about this. The patient is not keen to take medication and the GP is not keen to prescribe it. The man asks about referral to a sleep clinic and the GP explains that the local sleep clinic has a waiting list of over 1 year and that they are unable to see anyone that has not had a full workup and tried all the other possibilities first. They agree to meet again in 3 weeks to check on progress.

 KEY POINTS

- Insomnia is a common and debilitating condition that requires a full workup.
- There are many simple measures that can help.
- Referral to a sleep clinic is seldom required.

CASE 53: JOINT PAIN

History

A 51-year-old woman presents to her GP with a 2-month history of pain, swelling and stiffness in the finger joints and wrists of both hands. Her feet are also very painful and stiff when she first gets up in the morning. In fact, her symptoms are much worse when she wakes up and the stiffness takes at least an hour to pass. She has also been feeling unwell, tired, slightly feverish and just not her usual energetic self. She is perimenopausal and her periods, although less frequent, have been very heavy so she wonders if the symptoms might be menopausal in origin or whether she might be anaemic. She works as a dog walker and has been very busy recently so she wonders whether this might also be a factor and, it being winter, has been out in all weathers so has this got anything to do with it? She has been remarkably healthy up until now with no serious illnesses or operations. She is on no medication, apart from the occasional ibuprofen. On further questioning she has not had any rashes, eye problems, mouth ulcers, dry mouth, dry skin or hair, bowel disturbance or sensitivity to heat or cold. Her weight is stable. She appears bright and denies any depressive symptoms. She does not smoke and drinks about 10 units of alcohol per week. Her father died in a motor vehicle accident in his 40s and her mother, alive at 80 years, has hypothyroidism but is otherwise quite well. She does not know of any psoriasis in the family.

Examination

The patient looks well. The GP examines her hands, palms down with fingers straight, and her wrists. There does not appear to be any marked swelling or deformity although the patient says that her rings no longer come off because the finger joints are a bit swollen and the hands certainly are tender when the GP palpates them, especially when the metacarpal joints are squeezed. The movements of fingers and wrists are full. The GP looks carefully for a rash and cannot find one; there are no nail changes. The rest of the musculoskeletal examination is normal as is the cardiovascular, respiratory, abdominal and neurological examination. Her body mass index (BMI) is 24, as usual.

 INVESTIGATIONS

Urinalysis is normal apart from a trace of protein. The GP orders a full blood count, ferritin levels, erythrocyte sedimentation rate (ESR), C-reactive protein (CRP), renal function and autoantibodies, including rheumatoid factor. The results come back with a haemoglobin level of 11.4 g/dL, ferritin level on the lower side of normal, normal red cells, and a mildly elevated ESR of 13 mm/hour. All other results are normal.

Questions

- What is the differential diagnosis?
- What does the GP do next?

ANSWER

> The differential diagnosis includes rheumatoid arthritis; connective tissue diseases such as systemic lupus erythematosus (SLE); and osteoarthritis (with perimenopausal symptoms and mild anaemia, perhaps as a result of her menorrhagia). Gout usually affects one joint initially and there are no symptoms of a viral arthritis, one of the spondarthritides or psoriatic arthropathy.

With only mildly abnormal blood tests, the GP is inclined to prescribe some iron, repeat the blood tests in 6 weeks and see what happens, putting the symptoms down to perimenopausal symptoms. However, she has recently been to a general practice update on musculoskeletal medicine where it was said that early diagnosis and treatment of rheumatoid arthritis is essential to prevent progressive joint destruction and consequent impaired quality of life. This has got the GP worried. The patient certainly has the symptoms of rheumatoid arthritis with morning stiffness of over 1 hour, joint pain involving more than three joints, hand arthritis and symmetrical arthritis. Also, the patient is not one to complain or come to the GP unless really necessary. At the update they were told about a new test of antibodies to cyclic citrullinated peptides (anti-CCP) that can be present in rheumatoid arthritis where rheumatoid factor is absent.

The GP organizes for anti-CCP to be tested and it comes back positive. The GP arranges for an urgent referral to the rheumatologist who confirms a diagnosis of rheumatoid arthritis and starts the patient on the disease modifying anti-rheumatic drug (DMARD) methotrexate in association with folic acid. Regular monitoring of full blood count (FBC), liver function and urea and electrolytes is organized in tandem with the patient's general practice. The patient is also prescribed a non-steroidal anti-inflammatory drug (NSAID) for pain and stiffness in the hope that, once the DMARD starts working, the dose of the NSAID can be reduced. It is hoped that there will be a good response to the DMARD. If not, anti-tumour necrosis factor (anti-TNF) treatment will be instituted.

 KEY POINTS

- Rheumatoid arthritis is a common and destructive autoimmune disease affecting 1 per cent of the adult population and is three times as common in women as men. Be aware of the presenting symptoms.
- Early diagnosis and treatment is necessary to prevent joint destruction.
- Attend clinical updates and read medical literature to keep abreast of new developments in diagnosis and treatment.

CASE 54: LIFE EVENTS

History

The GP is visited by two new patients, a 65-year-old woman and her 67-year-old husband. They have recently moved into the area to be closer to their daughter. They tell the GP that they both have high blood pressure and have come for a check-up and for repeats of their medication. The woman also tells the doctor that she has arthritis in her lower back and her knees for which she takes paracetamol. Her husband reports that he has a high cholesterol and is on medication for this. Otherwise they say that they are reasonably well and have no other serious illness.

Examination

Brief examination reveals no other problems. However, they seem very sad, are not forthcoming about themselves and their situation and make little eye contact.

INVESTIGATIONS
The GP is concerned about them and arranges some blood tests and urinalyses with a follow-up appointment to see them with the results.

Questions

- Why is the GP concerned?
- How might the GP approach the situation?
- What is the outcome?

ANSWER

The GP is really concerned about their mental health. The physical problems of hypertension, arthritis and hypercholesterolaemia can be controlled with medication. However the GP notices that they are very sad and that they are finding it difficult to relate to her. Part of this is may be because they are new patients but there also appears to be something more going on. She has not elicited anything about their personal circumstances other than very basic information and does not yet have the old notes to refer to.

The GP would ordinarily repeat their medications and ask the practice nurse to follow up the investigations. However in this situation it is important for the GP to spend time with the new patients and build rapport and trust as they are in a vulnerable situation. She therefore organizes for the practice nurse to do the blood testing and for the patients to return to her for the results.

The GP continues to see the couple every few months for check-ups and review. They always come together and will not see the GP separately. She wonders whether there is something going on between them that they will not divulge when they are together. In the meantime their old notes arrive and the GP reads that, 20 years previously, they lost their only son to acquired immune deficiency syndrome (AIDS). Over time the couple talks more with the GP about themselves and about how their son's illness and death has affected them. They have tended to keep the reason for his death secret as they have felt shame about their son's demise. They admit to difficulties in their relationship but are not willing to open up more about this.

One day the GP gives the wife two creams: capsaicin cream for her sore back and oestrogen cream for her atrophic vaginitis. On giving her the prescription she advises her not to confuse the creams and explains what the results might be if she uses the capsaicin cream for her vaginitis. The patient finds this extremely funny and erupts into laughter, the first time she has laughed for many years. Her husband and the GP, surprised at first, join in. This is a turning point in the consultation and in the doctor–patient relationship. From this point the trust and rapport between the couple and the GP improves enormously. Nothing much changes; however, the GP feels that at least she can be there and act as a safety valve for the emotions and the difficulties that the couple experience.

 KEY POINTS

- Rapport and trust can take some time to develop.
- Continuity of care is the great strength of general practice.
- Sometimes very little can be done except to support and help patients by being there for them. This can make all the difference to a patient's quality of life.
- Be careful with humour: it can be helpful but can sometimes backfire badly.

CASE 55: LOIN PAIN

History

A 65-year-old woman consults her GP with a 1-day history of left-sided loin pain. The patient is accompanied by her husband; both are well known to the doctor. They are Italian and have lived in the UK for some years but their English is not fluent. The history is hard to elicit but with her husband's help it appears that the pain is aching in nature with sudden spasms of colicky pain that radiate around her abdomen and down into her groin. The pain meant that she had fitful sleep the night before. She has been passing urine a little more frequently than usual and did pass urine a few times in the night, which is unusual for her. She has no pain when she passes urine. Her urine has perhaps been a bit darker than usual and she feels nauseated and hot and cold. She appears to be in no particular pain as she is talking to you but grimaces and points to her back as she explains her symptoms. She often comes to her GP with aches and pains, some of which are related to osteoarthritis and others difficult to diagnose. The GP suspects a strong psychosomatic element to many of her ailments. She has a number of health problems including Type 2 diabetes mellitus, hypercholesterolaemia, and hypertension, all fairly well-controlled with medication although she is sedentary and enjoys cakes and fizzy drinks. She takes metformin 500 mg BD, simvastatin 40 mg daily and ramipril 1.25 mg daily. She has a long history of depression since the death of her daughter 15 years previously in a motor vehicle accident. Her husband is a little older than her, now retired having been a motor mechanic, and they have two other daughters, one of whom lives in London and the other in America. They live in a small, comfortable house that they own. Over the years her GP has developed a good relationship with them and recently the patient sometimes smiles and shares a funny story when they meet. However, her long history of depression has meant that it has been very hard for her and her husband to cope. She is not able to do anything around the house without her husband's help, even showering. She does cook but does not do the cleaning or shopping and a friend of hers comes around weekly to do this. Her husband gets very frustrated with this. Social services have been involved but she refuses to allow a home help in the house. She also refuses mental health assessment or treatment. Often when she has been referred for specialist care she does not attend or does not follow advice.

Questions
- What could be wrong with her?
- What does the GP do next?

ANSWER

> She may, once again, have symptoms that are indeterminate in nature, related to her sadness, and to which the GP cannot ascribe a physical illness. However, given that these symptoms are more specific and appear more painful than usual, the GP suspects a physical cause. The differential diagnosis would include renal colic, a urinary tract infection and a back problem.

The GP examines her and finds tenderness in the left loin and slight tenderness in the lower abdomen. The patient is afebrile. Blood pressure (BP) is normal at 136/80 mmHg and urinalysis reveals microscopic haematuria and a trace of protein, but is otherwise normal with no leucocytes or nitrites. There is nothing else to find on full examination; in particular examination of the patient's spine, although stiff, is normal. The patient has not had a past history of similar pain and has not suffered from recurrent urinary tract infections. The GP asks about family history of kidney stones but there is none. Renal calculi are more common in people with diabetes.

The GP sends off a urine for culture although the absence of nitrites and leucocytes makes infection unlikely. Blood is also taken for a full blood count, serum electrolytes and renal function although a blood test 6 months previously was normal for these tests. The GP also orders a plain abdominal X-ray as this will pick up renal stones that are radio-opaque. A computed tomography (CT) scan is the best test for the patient but the GP is unable to order this except through a urologist. The GP prescribes a short-term course of a non-steroidal anti-inflammatory drug (NSAID), diclofenac, in tablet form as the pain is not so severe as to indicate intramuscular injection or stronger pain relief, and asks the patient to drink plenty of fluids. The GP considers asking the patient to sieve her urine for stones but because of her psychological state and reluctance to engage, decides that this would not be possible and would just cause more conflict between the patient and her husband. A follow-up appointment is arranged for 1 week to monitor progress and the patient is advised to make an emergency appointment if the pain becomes worse. The GP explains that, if indeed the diagnosis is kidney stones, then the majority are passed within 1–3 weeks. Because of the patient's dislike of hospitals and doctors and the fact that this is her first attack, they decide to carry out simple investigations at this stage and, if the symptoms return, consider referral to a urologist.

 KEY POINTS

- It can be difficult to make diagnoses in patients who tend to somatize psychological problems and in such situations a doctor must always be aware that organic illness is still a possibility.
- It is important to communicate closely with patients and tailor expectations accordingly, working within what is possible.

History

The GP is visited by a 21-year-old woman who has just given birth. Her baby is now 2 weeks old and she has been seen previously by the community midwife. She seems very tired and quiet and the GP notices that she does not seem overly enthusiastic about her baby who is asleep. Her pregnancy was planned and was uneventful. She went into labour early and the baby was born at 36 weeks. Her labour was long and arduous and she needed a ventouse delivery as she was exhausted and the baby was distressed. The baby had a few days in the Special Care Baby Unit (SCBU) and was discharged from there in good health. She tells her GP that she tried to breast-feed but felt that the baby was not getting enough as he cried a lot and so she is now bottle-feeding. She lives with her partner who she has been with for the past 2 years and they have no other children. They live in a council flat and her partner works as a builder. She tells her GP that he has been very supportive. She works as a nursery assistant and is on maternity leave. Her mum and her sister live nearby and have been helping with the care of the baby. The patient has not had any previous physical or mental ill health. However, her father died suddenly and unexpectedly from a myocardial infarction the previous Christmas at the age of 60 years. She tells the GP that she feels low most of the time and is irritable with her partner and her family, which is not like her. She finds it hard to sleep. Her baby needs a feed at 10.30 p.m., 2.30 a.m. and 6.30 a.m. and her partner often does the 2.30 a.m. feed for her. She was very overweight and deliberately lost a lot of weight before she got pregnant. She is now 'comfort eating' and putting on weight again, which depresses her. She has not been interested in anything and not at all interested in sex, although she did have a large episiotomy and so she is still sore. She worries constantly that there is something wrong with her baby or that something bad will happen and finds it difficult to bond with the baby.

Questions

- What should the GP be concerned about?
- What would the GP need to find out?
- What could be done to help the patient and her baby?

ANSWER

The GP would be concerned about the possibility of postnatal depression or even puerperal psychosis. There are a number of risk factors which include a difficult delivery, a premature baby who needed care in the SCBU, and the recent death of her father. The GP, very early on in the consultation, realizes that this consultation is going to take time. As her appointment is near the end of the surgery the GP asks her to wait a little while so that the other two patients can be seen and more time can be given to her appointment. The GP explores how she is feeling. Mostly she just feels terribly guilty and sad that she is not enjoying her baby as she thought she would. She knows that she is not well and feels too ashamed to tell her family how she feels and worried that she will not cope and the baby will be taken away from her. The GP notices that, although she is very down, she is in touch with reality, she is aware that she is not well and she expresses herself clearly. Her GP asks her to complete the Edinburgh Postnatal Depression Scale (EPDS). In particular, the GP is keen to know whether the mother has had thoughts of harming herself. She scores 18 out of 30 but has not felt like harming herself. The GP diagnoses postnatal depression (PND).

The woman is very relieved that her distress has been recognized and that she has had the courage to tell the GP how she has been feeling. Her GP explains that PND is common, with about one in ten woman suffering from the condition, and that it needs treatment or the suffering can last for months and undermine her relationship with her baby as well as her partner. They talk about the factors that might have contributed to this situation and what can be done to help. She agrees to talk with her family and to come back the next day with her partner to talk about the next steps. The GP makes contact with the health visitor (with the patient's permission). She also makes contact with the local mental health organization, which has a specialist service for postnatal depression. The patient enters into counselling and is also put onto an antidepressant.

 KEY POINTS

- For important consultations, such as this, give your patient and yourself time to explore the issues.
- Over 50 per cent of women with postnatal depression are missed by GPs and health visitors.
- Research is growing that untreated PND damages the psychological development of the young child and that there is also an increase in depression in the partner, thus compounding the problems.
- It is important to be aware of the possibility of severe mental health problems in all new mothers, whether or not there are predisposing factors.

CASE 57: MALAISE

History

A 16-year-old school girl returns to the surgery with her mother. One week previously she had been seen by the nurse practitioner and was diagnosed with acute tonsillitis. The nurse practitioner noted a history of sore throat with swallowing difficulties, severe malaise, muscle aches all over the body, shivering, swelling around the eyes and headaches. The examination revealed a temperature of 39.6°C, severe pharyngitis, reddened, purulent and enlarged tonsils, a puffiness of the upper eyelids; and cervical lymphadenopathy. The nurse practitioner prescribed a 7-day course of penicillin V and advised the patient to increase her fluid intake, rest and take regular paracetamol.

The mother is concerned because her daughter has not recovered. At first the antibiotics seemed to help and the temperature, sore throat and headaches improved. After 4 days the eye swelling had disappeared, but on the next day a faint non-itchy red rash developed. The mother thought it might be a 'mild allergy' to the penicillin, but they decided to continue treatment as long the rash did not worsen. While the pain in the throat is better, the patient complains of more pains in her neck and the recurrence of headaches. The worst symptom of all is the total lack of energy and mother is concerned that her daughter sleeps 18 hours a day: 'That is so unusual for Linda, something else must be wrong with her'. The young woman is concerned about not having the energy to study for her upcoming GCSEs.

Examination

On examination she looks pale, unwell and exhausted with a slightly yellowy sclera. Her temperature is 37.6°C. There are multiple swollen and tender lymph nodes palpable in the anterior and posterior cervical regions, bilaterally. Her throat is still inflamed, and the tonsils enlarged, but without white patches. There is a faint red macular rash all over her trunk spreading to the limbs. The tip of the spleen is palpable on deep inspiration, the liver palpable and mildly tender, and swollen lymph nodes are also found in both axillae and inguinal fossae.

Questions
- What is the diagnosis and differential diagnosis?
- What tests if any would you initiate?
- What advice would you give the patient?

ANSWER

Glandular fever is the most likely diagnosis. The initial diagnosis of acute tonsillitis by the nurse practitioner was reasonable. Acute tonsillitis is seen far more commonly in primary care and would have been a disease susceptible to antibiotic treatment although the rash may have been triggered by the antibiotic or may be from the illness itself. The further list of potential diagnoses is long and includes acute *Human immunodeficiency virus* (HIV) infection, diphtheria, toxoplasmosis, cytomegalovirus and leukaemia.

The Paul–Bunnell reaction (Monospot) – heterophile immunoglobulin M (IgM) antibodies agglutinating sheep erythrocytes – is the most commonly used screening test for glandular fever. It can be falsely negative, especially in young patients, or falsely positive, for example owing to cytomegalovirus. A full blood count should show a leucocytosis between 10 000 and 20 000 cells/mm^3, thrombocytopenia (often), and on the blood film many atypical activated T-lymphocytes (mononucleosis cells). More than 20 per cent atypical lymphocytes or more than 50 per cent lymphocytes with at least 10 per cent atypical lymphocytes on blood film make the diagnosis very likely. There are more specific immunological tests for Epstein–Barr virus available which can be useful if the Paul–Bunnell test is negative. Glandular fever (infectious mononucleosis, or kissing disease) is an infection of the B-lymphocytes by the Epstein–Barr virus. It is a self-limiting disease that in young children often goes unnoticed, but in young adults causes glandular fever. The virus is secreted in the saliva and can be transmitted through close bodily contact (kissing) or sharing utensils (cups, cutlery, towels). The incubation period is 4–8 weeks. Most patient recover within 2 weeks with some residual tiredness for another week. However, a significant minority go on to suffer with tiredness for much longer.

The patient presents with all the clinical signs of glandular fever and does not need any further testing. However, it can be reassuring to the patient and relatives to have the diagnosis confirmed, especially as her initial diagnosis differed. She needs to avoid contact sport because of the potential for damage to her swollen spleen, for 1–2 months. She should see herself as infectious while she is feeling unwell, avoiding sharing utensils and close bodily contact. She should rest and expect to start feeling better after 2 weeks, being back to normal energy levels at around 4 weeks.

 KEY POINTS

- Early presentations of disease can be deceptive, with the correct diagnosis emerging later in its progression.
- Proper diagnosis and sensible advice are reassuring for the patient and their family, whether or not there is effective medical treatment.

History

A 53-year-old chief executive returns early to his GP for his hypertension review. Since he and his wife had read an article in *The Guardian* about the ASCOT Trial reporting that a 'drug switch can cut the risk of heart attack by half' his wife has been asking him to go to the doctor and have his medications changed. The GP responds by looking through the patient's records. The patient initially presented with raised blood pressure 8 years ago. At this time his untreated blood pressure was around 170/95 mmHg on several occasions; there was no family history of ischaemic heart disease, stroke or diabetes, his body mass index (BMI) was 28, he never smoked and his alcohol intake was 50 units per week. He went to the gym twice a week and had a well-balanced diet. His total fasting cholesterol was 6.1 mmol/L and his fasting blood glucose was normal. At that time he was not keen to start on medication and so he received lifestyle advice from the practice nurse, who asked him to reduce his alcohol and salt intake, reduce his weight and increase his exercise. At a 6-month review his blood pressure had not improved and so he agreed to start on atenolol at a dose of 50 mg daily. He responded well to the medication, with no side-effects, and his blood pressure dropped to around 145/90 mmHg. At the next review the doctor added bendroflumethiazide at a dose of 2.5 mg daily and his blood pressure dropped further to 125/80 mmHg. Six-monthly reviews since have documented a consistently well-controlled blood pressure, while the patient maintains his slightly raised BMI and cholesterol.

Having established the past medical history the GP asks the patient what his concerns are. The patient replies that his wife tells him that GPs use old-fashioned tablets such as diuretics and beta-blockers to save money and that these tablets cause diabetes. His wife feels that he is already at risk of diabetes because he is overweight. He denies erectile dysfunction. The article said that the newer and more expensive angiotensin-converting enzyme (ACE)-inhibitors and calcium channel blockers reduce the risk of cardiovascular death by 25 per cent compared with the old medications and that this risk is reduced even further if the cholesterol-lowering drug atorvastatin is added in. The patient then pulls out a folder of cuttings from the newspapers and printouts from the internet: 'I think you will find it all in here, doctor. Could you please change my tablets and start me on atorvastatin?'

Questions

- Should the GP change the blood pressure medication as requested by the patient?
- How would you decide whether to add atorvastatin?
- Assuming that you agree to change the patient's medication is there anything you would like to warn the patient about?
- What do you think will be the emotional response of the GP faced with this situation?
- Should GPs always change patients' treatments when new evidence emerges?

Guidelines for the treatment of chronic disease are continuously updated. Doctors have a duty to keep their knowledge up to date but often clinical studies get into the headlines before they are translated to guidelines. The patient is making a reasonable request for updating his treatment. It would be reasonable to expect that the GP checks the latest edition of the *British National Formulary* for guidance.

In order to increase adherence to treatment it is good practice for doctors, in consultation with the patient, to establish a treatment plan. The patient's interest in their medication can then be seen positively, allowing them to own the treatment decisions of their condition. While there is good evidence for cholesterol-lowering treatment for secondary prophylaxis for patients with cardiovascular disease, there is no convincing evidence for statins for primary prophylaxis. However, it has become common practice to offer statins as primary prophylaxis for patients who have an increased risk for cardiovascular disease (CVD). There is no convincing evidence showing the superiority of one statin above another and so the GP should choose the cheapest option.

The GP will be concerned that the requested treatments might not yield the same therapeutic success as that achieved with the current medication. A shift of medication will necessitate a period when the patient's blood pressure response will need to be monitored and if an ACE-inhibitor is used each dose change requires a kidney function blood test. The patient should be informed of all this as well as possible side-effects and be encouraged to report back if they arise.

Many GPs will feel their heart sink when faced with a patient attending with a thick file of paper cuttings and internet printouts, and requesting a change of medication. The GP might feel threatened by the knowledge that the patient brings to the consultation and afraid to be 'found out' about not being up to date on the topic. Other GPs might feel undervalued by the patient for the good care that they have provided in treating the blood pressure successfully. They might fear that changing the treatment will 'rock the boat', leaving the patient with a less well-controlled blood pressure and the possibility that they themselves will be out of pocket if the treatment targets for the Quality and Outcomes Framework (QOF) cannot be achieved.

It is important that GPs have systems in place to identify and recall patients when new prescribing evidence emerges. The ASCOT study showed only marginally improved absolute risk reduction for patients treated with the more modern drug combination. It took some time before national guidelines incorporated the findings, and many patients chose to continue on their old drug regimes, avoiding the upheaval of changing treatments.

 KEY POINTS

- Doctors should aim to establish treatment plans in consultation with their patients.
- Patient access to medical knowledge has improved markedly with the introduction of the internet.
- New evidence can be available to patients before it has been translated into GP guidelines.

History

Your next patient is a 45-year-old businessman, a property dealer with a city office and a comfortable home. He is accustomed to making trips back to India, where his parents and extended family still live. He has come today for a routine blood pressure (BP) check and prescription before another visit. He says that his father suffers from asthma, and has been advised by his doctor in India to use a particular brand of bronchodilator, which is not easily available over there. He would like you to give him a prescription, in his name, so that he can take supplies out to his father. He says other doctors have given him such prescriptions in the past.

Questions

- What reasons have you for declining this request?
- Can you offer treatment privately instead?

ANSWER

The services of the NHS are freely available to anyone resident in the UK. This includes any visitor from abroad, for emergency care. There are reciprocal agreements with the governments of many countries in Europe, but not with most of the Commonwealth, or with the USA or most of Africa or Asia. If a registered patient travels abroad, you may prescribe a reasonable quantity of their own drugs for personal use – a couple of months of his own hypotensive would be acceptable. But this privilege does not extend to residents of other countries: the NHS cannot accept the burden of health care for anyone in the world. Furthermore, you may not treat a patient for whom you do not have clinical responsibility. At the very least, you must have seen and examined the patient, and be in a position to do the same again when needed. So it is impossible for you to issue a prescription in his father's name, either NHS or private. Writing the prescription in the patient's own name would be improper behaviour, which could lead to your facing a stricture from the General Medical Council. If the medication is not marked in the *British National Formulary* as 'POM' (Prescription-only Medicine) he may be able to buy it from a chemist over the counter, but will need to check with the airline whether he can carry it in his luggage. If he brings his father to the UK, you must point out that he would still not be entitled to NHS treatment, as his pre-existing condition would not be classed as an emergency. Whether you could treat him as a private patient would depend on your practice's policy regarding such care; it is a good idea to ensure your practice has a protocol for such situations, drawn up with the guidance of your medical insurance advisers, and your local primary care trust. In this case, he is disappointed at your refusal.

If his trip is likely to be more that a couple of months, you may offer to give him a letter, summarizing his own current medical state, and listing his own treatment: he will need to get more supplies of his medication while he is abroad, and he should be warned that he may face the same supply difficulties that his father is experiencing, as UK treatments are by no means widely available worldwide; don't forget to remind him to keep his travel immunizations up to date, and to take his antimalarials.

 KEY POINTS

- Be aware of entitlement for treatment for overseas visitors and NHS patients seeking treatment abroad. This information can be found on the Department of Health website.
- A doctor prescribing a medication bears responsibility for that treatment and must know the patient and the patient's condition and be able to follow up the treatment outcomes.

CASE 60: MULTIPLE SYMPTOMS

History

The computer record for the next patient shows a warning box: 'Fat notes'. The old Lloyd George paper records are stuffed into two bulky envelopes, and tell a story of many consultations with GP, and hospital, over the years. Symptoms such as backache, headache, dizziness, weakness, cough, fill the pages and no clear diagnosis emerges, apart from vague labels such as 'neurasthenia', 'supra-tentorial' and 'psychosomatic'. Meeting her for the first time, she appears a slightly vague woman, who gives a rambling history of indigestion, aches and pains, constipation, swollen legs, and so on. She is 44 years old, married, with one daughter at school. Her present symptoms have been troubling her 'for some time', which could be weeks or months.

Examination

It is traditional to start by taking the pulse. In her case, it is regular, but a surprising 40 beats/minute. Her blood pressure is 140/85 mmHg, her skin feels cool and dry, and she has bilateral rather indurated leg oedema, with some reddening of the skin.

 INVESTIGATIONS

Her full blood count, blood glucose, renal and liver function tests are normal. Her fasting cholesterol level is 6.5 mmol/L.

Questions
- What other aspects of examination would you like to know about?
- Are further tests indicated, and if so, what?

ANSWER

She has no goitre; her tendon reflexes are difficult to assess. Her thyroid function test returns with a high thyroid-stimulating hormone (TSH) level, and a very low free thyroxine: a clear case of hypothyroidism. The laboratory reports on her thyroglobulin antibodies, supporting the diagnosis of primary hypothyroidism. An electrocardiogram (ECG) shows low-voltage bradycardia.

You start treatment with 25 μg of levothyroxine daily, rising slowly, step-wise, to 100 μg. The transformation is remarkable. In a month, she becomes alert and active, with bright eyes; she loses 2 kg in weight and smartens her hairstyle and her clothing. She still has a list of problems, but she is no longer constipated or oedematous.

National Health Service guidance suggests referral for the following groups with this condition:

- under 16 years of age;
- pregnant or postpartum;
- have particular management problems (e.g. coronary heart disease, on amiodarone or lithium);
- where TSH level fails to return to normal, despite a dose of 200 μg or more of levothyroxine;
- continue to be symptomatic, despite apparently adequate levothyroxine replacement.

This patient will need lifelong thyroxine replacement therapy, with measurement of TSH at least annually to check compliance and that the dose is still correct. She should be encouraged to apply for free prescriptions on the NHS, for this and all other conditions in the future.

 KEY POINTS

- One of the charms of general practice is the slight frisson of uncertainty before the door opens for each patient. Even the most familiar 'friend' could turn out to have a new illness this time.
- When facing a 'heart-sink' patient with a familiar litany, try to listen to the tale with fresh ears and an unbiased mind; you might discover something new this time.
- Be careful that your notes are respectful: comments such as 'supra-tentorial' are not acceptable.

CASE 61: MUSCLE PAIN

History

The GP is visited by his patient, a 65-year-old woman, who had been diagnosed as having adhesive capsulitis of the right shoulder some months previously (see Case 85). The GP had referred her for physiotherapy to stretch the muscles and restore function and mobility, and she had taken simple paracetamol for pain relief. This had helped and the pain was less troublesome and the range of movements had increased although the patient was aware that it could take some time for her to recover substantially. Also of importance was that she had received some bereavement counselling from Cruse Bereavement Care and she had found this very helpful (see Case 85). She has been visiting the GP regularly and feeling much more hopeful about things. She was even managing to get out and about more; she has been food shopping, going to bingo once a week and having her friends around for coffee. Apart from her shoulder problem her health has been good and physical examination and blood tests (full blood count, renal, liver, thyroid and lipid profiles and blood glucose) have all been normal. She is on no other medication apart from the paracetamol.

She tells the GP that, over the past 2-3 weeks, she has been suffering from general pain and stiffness, particularly in her thighs and both shoulders. Her GP is tempted to put this down to her sadness and isolation as well as lack of exercise owing to her sore shoulder and fear of going outside since she was mugged (see Case 85). However, the GP asks the patient to explain her symptoms in more detail. She reports that these symptoms started quite suddenly and that, in the morning when she wakes up, she has really bad and painful generalized stiffness, making it hard to move and that this stiffness lasts for at least an hour before easing. It makes it particularly hard for her to walk up and down stairs and raise her good arm to get dressed. After sitting for any length of time the stiffness also becomes a real problem. She is not feeling very well, has lost some weight and sometimes even feels that she is running a bit of a fever. She has not had any recent respiratory tract or other infection and has not been suffering from headaches. At times the symptoms wake her at night and prevent her from turning over in bed.

Questions

- What is the differential diagnosis?
- What other questions and examination should the GP focus on?
- What investigations might help?

ANSWER

The most probable diagnosis is this patient's case is polymyalgia rheumatica (PMR). Other possibilities are rheumatoid arthritis or other connective tissue disease, multiple myeloma and depression.

The GP should enquire about and carry out a full examination of the musculoskeletal system, particularly palpating the muscles for signs of tenderness, palpating the temporal muscles to look for temporal arteritis and examining the peripheral joints for any synovitis. Investigations will include a full blood count, erythrocyte sedimentation rate (ESR), C-reactive protein (CRP, usually raised with PMR) and liver function test (may be raised alkaline phosphatase with PMR). In this case the GP is fairly certain the diagnosis is PMR as the woman is in the right age group, has muscle tenderness in the upper arms, prolonged morning stiffness, an acute illness and weight loss. If the GP is not certain, additional tests can include protein electrophoresis to exclude a myeloma, and rheumatoid factor and antinuclear antibody to look for rheumatoid arthritis or other connective tissue disease. The patient's erythrocyte sedimentation rate (ESR) comes back at 50 mm/hour and her CRP at 10 mg/L. After speaking on the phone with the local rheumatologist the GP starts her on 15 mg prednisolone a day, which brings rapid relief of symptoms within a few days. Over the next 18 months she continues on a tapering dose of steroids and her blood tests revert to normal. She is put on weekly bisphosphonates to prevent osteoporosis, as should all patients over 65 years of age who are on steroids for over 3 months.

 KEY POINTS

- Multiple pathologies can occur.
- Do not blame everything on depression.
- A trial of medication is sometimes a very useful diagnostic tool.
- Watch out for iatrogenic disease.

CASE 62: MUSCLE PAIN

History

A 58-year-old builder attends the surgery with generalized joint and muscle pains and weakness of his proximal muscles. He is unable to get up from a lying position in bed, having to roll over onto his front to push himself up, and he has problems getting up from the sofa. The muscle pain and weakness have been slowly getting worse over the last 5 years. The ankles, knees and wrists are painful at all times and he has increasing difficulty in doing his work. He is feeling very exhausted and tired, his mood is low and he becomes irritable very easily. He has been crying unprovoked. He admits to problems falling asleep at night and early-morning waking. He has daily thoughts of life not being worth living, but denies any suicidal thoughts or intent. He has suffered two bereavements recently: a good friend dying after a short illness and the death of his father-in-law, to whom he was very close. He had an episode of depression 7 years previously when his business was in severe trouble and he responded well to antidepressant medication at that time.

The computer records show that he has been treated for essential hypertension with atenolol 50 mg once daily and enalapril 10 mg once daily for the last 6 years and for familial hypercholesterolaemia with simvastatin 40 mg at night (the dose increased 3 months ago). He was found to have raised blood pressure after an episode of non-cardiac chest pain and routine investigations revealed his raised cholesterol levels. Treatment for his hypercholesterolaemia was started because his 10-year coronary heart disease (CHD) and stroke risks were raised above the threshold for treatment.

🔍 INVESTIGATIONS

Recent observations and tests are as follows:

Blood pressure (BP):	138/84 mmHg
Body mass index (BMI):	31.2
Normal kidney function including eGFR	
Total cholesterol:	5.3 mmol/L
Serum triglycerides:	3.7 mmol/L
Normal serum creatine kinase (CK) level	
Fasting glucose:	6.5 mmol/L
Normal liver function tests	
Erythrocyte sedimentation rate (ESR):	13 mm/hour

Normal full blood count (FBC)
His PHQ-9 score is 23 (see Table 62.1).

Table 62.1 Over the last 2 weeks, how often have you been bothered by any of the following problems?

	Not at all	Several days	More than half the days	Nearly every day
Little interest or pleasure in doing things?				3
Feeling down, depressed, or hopeless?				3
Trouble falling or staying asleep, or sleeping too much?				3
Feeling tired or having little energy?				3
Poor appetite or overeating?		1		
Feeling bad about yourself – or that you are a failure or have let yourself or your family down?				3
Trouble concentrating on things, such as reading the newspaper or watching television?			2	
Moving or speaking so slowly that other people could have noticed?				
Or the opposite – being so fidgety or restless that you have been moving around a lot more than usual?			2	
Thoughts that you would be better off dead, or of hurting yourself in some way?				3

Questions

- What are his medical problems?
- How would you treat his problems?

ANSWER

- *Myalgia associated with statin treatment*: about 5 per cent of patients on statins complain of muscle pains. The myotoxicity is a function of the drug dose rather then low-density lipoprotein-cholesterol reduction. The HMG-CoA (3-hydroxy-3-methylglutaryl coenzyme A) reductase inhibitor reduces the production of the intermediates of cholesterol synthesis, which are utilized in the manufacture of ubiquinone, essential for electron transport in mitochondria. Patients with underlying muscle disorders, hypothyroidism, renal impairment, alcohol abuse or taking concomitant lipid-lowering or certain other drugs are at higher risk. This patient suffered with muscle pains ever since he started on statin treatment. The last increase in treatment aggravated his symptoms. The normal CK level excludes more severe myopathies.
- *Severe depressive episode*: a PHQ-9 score above 20 is considered to signal a severe episode of depression. Depression is an episodic long-term illness and the previous episode makes the diagnosis more likely, with the patient more likely to accept the diagnosis. It is impossible to decide whether his physical symptoms have made his depression worse or the other way around. However, the pain has made it more difficult for him to do his job and his business has begun to suffer. Previous business problems set off his first episode of depression and are likely to remain a strong trigger. This patient has lost two close friends over a short period of time increasing his vulnerability to develop a mood disorder. Patients with mood disorders must be assessed for their risk to self-harm or commit suicide.
- *Metabolic syndrome (Syndrome-X)*: metabolic syndrome is a cluster of conditions that, when they occur together, signal a high risk for CHD, stroke and diabetes. This patient has hypertension, raised cholesterol and triglyceride levels, impaired glucose tolerance and is obese. None of these conditions produce any symptoms and patients do not feel ill. The treatment aim is to reduce the risk of developing future disease.

The doctor stops the simvastatin. Over the next few weeks the muscle pain and weakness reduce significantly and 6 months later the symptoms have completely resolved. The patient is offered talking therapies, and bereavement counselling. However, he prefers antidepressant medication that had helped in the previous episode, understanding that treatment would need to be continued for at least 6 months. The medication initially caused nausea, but he persevered and his mood started to improve after 2 weeks. Eight months later he is reducing the medication successfully. The treatment for metabolic syndrome has two parts: modifying lifestyle and medication to treat lipids, high blood glucose and blood pressure. This patient's next fasting glucose was above the threshold for diagnosing diabetes. Feeling physically and mentally better, the new diagnosis motivated him to tackle his lifestyle issues with diet and exercise. Repeated blood tests showed reducing cholesterol levels, precluding the need for further treatment.

 KEY POINTS

- It is important to watch out for unwanted medication effects.
- Patients need to be assisted holistically.
- Lifestyle issues are tackled more easily by patients when they are psychologically well.

CASE 63: NECK SWELLING

History
Your next patient is a 35-year-old Afro-Caribbean woman who is complaining of a swelling in her neck. Keeping in mind the six basic questions (what, why, when, how, where and who), you establish that it has been present for a few weeks and is painless. She does not volunteer any other symptoms but seems not quite as well as you might expect. She has tried to lose weight, and after years of failure has achieved a loss of about 4.5 kg in the last 3 months. She says her asthma (she uses a salbutamol inhaler) has been troubling her during the summer months, and her legs are swelling. She does not admit to fever or malaise.

Examination
She has a firm, non-tender, slightly irregular mass about the size of a walnut situated in the front of her neck to the left, just above the collarbone. The lump does not move on swallowing and it is not tender. It feels solid and has no bruit. You are not sure if the neighbouring lymph glands are palpable or not as the patient is rather plump. You ask to examine her chest, which sounds a little more wheezy than usual. She consents to a breast examination, declining a chaperone, which reveals no tumours or other signs of malignancy. Her legs are somewhat obese, a little oedematous, and she has tender red bumps on her shins. There are no other positive signs on a general examination.

	INVESTIGATIONS
	You ask for a chest X-ray, which shows bilateral hilar lymphadenopathy.

Questions
- What are the likely differential diagnoses?
- What do you do next?

ANSWERS

Faced with a wide variety of diagnoses, you could use a 'surgical sieve' to try to reduce the possibilities to manageable proportions. Two that are popular are:

- VANISHED: Vascular, Accident, Neoplastic, Inflammatory, 'Septic' (i.e. infectious), Haematological or Hereditary, Endocrine, Degenerative
- VITAMIN D: Vascular, Infectious, Traumatic, Autoimmune, Metabolic, Inflammatory, Neoplastic, Degenerative.

Some categories can be eliminated quickly: there is no history of trauma; the lump does not move on swallowing, so it is not thyroid tissue; it is not tender, so is unlikely to be an acute infection; it feels solid, and has no bruit, so a vascular malformation is not the cause.

The differential diagnosis seems to lie between a neoplasm, an inflammatory disorder or a chronic infection. The swollen shins are probably erythema nodosum.

Prompt referral to the chest clinic results in her starting a course of steroids for sarcoidosis, a condition more common in women and in the Afro-Caribbean population. When she returns to you, you reinforce that this is a chronic condition, which will require such treatment from time to time, but is compatible with a long and active life (the overall mortality is reported as less than 3 per cent). Cooperating with the chest clinic, you arrange to monitor her weight and blood pressure (both likely to rise with the steroids), and check her full blood count and renal function.

 KEY POINTS

- Mnemonics are the last resort of the desperate – which is why we all use them sometimes. Keep them few, keep them short and keep them memorable.
- Thinking clearly and logically is, however, essential.
- Some illnesses do not fall neatly into the artificial categories of a list. If it is not obvious, be prepared to think 'outside the box'.
- Unexplained weight loss is a 'red-flag' symptom, and should trigger a referral for further investigation; the problem sometimes is to determine to which speciality.

History

The GP is about to make a follow-up phone call to the patient of Case 37. Three weeks ago, receiving the results of the chest X-ray, he started the patient on amoxicillin and arranged a repeat chest X-ray. With the long smoking history in mind and the history of increasing muscle weakness, probably caused by a paraneoplastic phenomenon, he decided not to await the X-ray results, but initiated a referral to the chest clinic under the 2-week rule for suspected lung cancer. The patient was told about the suspected diagnosis and the possible alternative infective causes. Sputum investigations had been arranged and had come back normal.

The GP had visited the patient once because of increasing weakness and confusion, predominantly at night. The patient had been complaining of a productive cough and on examination the doctor found a raised temperature of 38.2°C, tachypnoea and crepitation over the left upper areas, but the patient seemed to be lucid. The GP changed the antibiotic treatment to clarithromycin. Three days previously the surgery had received a fax from the chest clinic confirming the diagnosis of lung cancer. Unfortunately, the disease involved large areas of the lung and the oncologist judged that curative treatment was futile. The letter stated that, as the patient was having no symptoms, he needed no palliative treatment at the moment, but that radiation treatment would be available if he developed pain, dyspnoea or bleeding.

The GP gets through to the wife first. She tells him that the patient is much improved: 'He has been out in the yard all by himself for the first time in a year. The hospital doctor told us there is no cure, and I'm so worried about him. He won't speak to me about it'. She hands the phone over to her husband. 'Doctor, I don't understand what is happening. After you referred me to the chest clinic I was seen the following week. The consultant did all his tests and I had to return to see a nurse who discharged me after offering me some cough linctus. I don't seem to have any follow-up appointments for treatment'.

Questions
- How should the GP respond?
- Why does the patient seem not to be aware of his terminal diagnosis?

ANSWER

The patient seems to be confused about his illness. The GP needs to arrange a face-to-face meeting with the patient and it would be inappropriate to continue the telephone consultation at this point. The meeting could take place in the surgery or at the patient's home. A meeting in the surgery would save the doctor's time and could be seen as more efficient. A home visit, however, would allow the doctor to avoid work interruptions and show appreciation for the patient's autonomy, increasing the likelihood that the patient will feel confident enough to speak up and ask his questions. It is not surprising for the patient to be confused. Within a very short period of time he has received several diagnoses, some of which have turned out to be wrong. After a long and slow decline of his strength, climaxing in a fall causing him to stay a night on the floor, he was given hope by being placed on steroids. When the antibiotic treatment failed to cure his condition, the results of the abnormal chest X-ray arrived. The new referral guidelines for suspected malignancies allowed him to be tracked through the system rapidly, giving an impression of urgency. The patient might have still been considering his diagnosis of lung cancer when he was given the news that his illness had progressed beyond curative treatment – since he was not suffering from any specific chest symptoms, this news might have been even less comprehensible.

 KEY POINTS

- Informing patients of their diagnosis does not necessarily mean that they have heard it, understood it or the treatment options that follow.
- Breaking bad news is a process that in some cases needs to be spread over time.

History

The next patient consults with the GP frequently. The list of problems on the computer runs to three pages; the old paper record has similarly three full envelopes. She has variously been diagnosed with anxiety, depression, hypochondriasis, mild personality disorder, globus hystericus, as well as Type I diabetes, chronic bronchitis, and recurrent urinary infections. She is now 62 years old, married, with two grown sons. Today, she has come to see you with pain 'here' and 'here', and 'here', pointing to her epigastrium, right loin, and sternum, respectively. You ask if her regular medication, omeprazole, is helping and she emphatically says 'no'. She also gains little relief from alginate mixture.

Examination

Examination is singularly unhelpful, since she is so obese that you cannot distinguish any abdominal landmarks. You note she has had endoscopy in the past, which did confirm reflux oesophagitis.

Questions

- What other information might be useful here?
- What would your priorities be in her further care?

ANSWER

Routine enquiry shows that she smokes about 30 cigarettes a day, but drinks rarely. Her diabetes is erratically controlled, her latest glycated haemoglobin being 13.4 per cent. You temporize by arranging a urine test, and adjusting her insulin dose. You also ask for a fasting lipid profile and renal and thyroid function tests.

An opportunity arises a few days later to see her husband, who is chronically depressed. He reveals that he is desperately worried about their finances. Their home is on its second mortgage, and they cannot meet the repayments, and it is likely to be repossessed. This is surprising, since they had been comfortably off in the past. It appears that his wife is a gambler, spending all and more of their money at casinos. Her behaviour has driven away her sons, who have rejected her. Her husband has thought of divorce, but is still fond of her and does not wish to desert her.

You suggest she might contact Gamblers Anonymous, but he says she doesn't admit to any problem. You give him information about the family support group, Gam-Anon. When you next see her you try to explore some of this background but she is scathing about her husband's inability to provide for her, and about her ungrateful sons. You adjust her proton-pump prescription, monitor her inhalers, and ask her to see the diabetes nurse. You arrange to see her again in 1 month.

 KEY POINTS

- With the best will in the world, some patients resist attempts to help them. In this case, you may be restricted to damage limitation, and to maintaining contact with her over a period of time, in case she gains enough trust in you to listen to your advice.
- Gambling can be even more destructive to families than alcohol, and is worth bearing in mind as a possible cause if a family appears under strain.

History

The GP is visited by a 61-year-old Afro-Caribbean woman. She seldom visits the practice and the last time the GP had seen her was some months previously when she had brought her grandchild in with a sore ear. She has been remarkably healthy and vigorous and so the GP is shocked by her appearance. She is downcast and moving slowly, and eases herself down into the chair in the consulting room with a sigh, shaking her head. The GP enquires what the matter is and she reports that she has pain all over her body and feels very tired and that this has been going on for the past month. She points to her head, her shoulders her back and abdomen as well as her knees and feet. On questioning her further with regard to her physical condition there appear to be no other symptoms. She has not wanted to bother the doctor but her family has persuaded her to attend.

She has no past medical history of note and her weight and blood pressure have always been within normal limits. She does not have sickle cell trait or sickle cell disease and is on no medication apart from the occasional paracetamol that she takes for minor aches and pains.

The patient grew up in Jamaica and came to England in the 1950s. She married and she and her husband, who worked for British Telecom, brought up their five children in West London. Her husband was much older than her and had died 5 years previously from coronary artery disease. She now lives in a council house that she shares with her youngest daughter and her daughter's four children who are aged 10, 7, 5 and 1 year. Her daughter works as a receptionist in a local dental surgery and the patient helps look after the household. Her four other children all live nearby and they are a close and supportive family. She always has grandchildren around her and is the bedrock of the family.

Questions
- How does the GP approach the consultation with this patient?
- What examination and investigations are appropriate?
- What is the outcome?

ANSWER

The GP takes a careful history and does a full examination, covering all the systems, focusing particularly on the neurological and musculoskeletal system. Apart from the patient wincing when any of her muscles are palpated there are no other signs or symptoms of note. There is no temporal tenderness. There is no stiffness or weakness and no particular joint stiffness or swelling. There are no skin problems, no lymphadenopathy and breast examination is normal. She has not had any recent illness and her weight is stable. Her bowels and urine (including urinalysis) are normal. She is not on any regular medication, in particular a statin. When the GP talks with her further it transpires that her son's wife recently had a stillborn child. The couple had many problems conceiving and this was their first child. The patient tells the doctor also of the miscarriage that she had when still a young woman, new in the UK and without family around her.

The doctor feels almost certain that her symptoms are a somatic response to her sadness. He talks with the patient about this and she is amenable to the possibility. However there is a small chance that the symptoms could be caused by a physical illness, for example polymyalgia rheumatica, thyroid disease, systemic lupus erythematosus, or a malignancy or even vitamin D deficiency. The GP therefore orders some blood tests including full blood count (FBC), erythrocyte sedimentation rate (ESR), C-reactive protein (CRP), autoantibody screen, rheumatoid factor, vitamin D levels, thyroid, liver and renal function. As she is having blood taken the GP also orders fasting lipids and blood glucose. These come back normal, making any of these physical diagnoses unlikely.

 KEY POINTS

- It is important to think carefully about possible diagnoses and probabilities, minimizing medicalization and investigation.
- Somatization is a common disorder, reported in many cultures, particularly as manifestation of sadness and unhappiness.
- The pattern of somatization can differ in different cultures and it is worthwhile having an understanding of this, particularly as this affects the cultural backgrounds of your patients.
- Don't forget about vitamin D deficiency: it can cause symptoms such as aches and pains, is estimated to be present in two out of ten adults in the UK, and is more common in people with dark skins.

History

A 24-year-old man sees his GP, complaining that his tongue stings when he eats spicy food. The discomfort has developed over the last 3 weeks. At first he thought that he had eaten too much spicy food and 'burned' his tongue. He looked at his tongue and found red areas. Much to his concern the red areas have moved.

Looking through his health records the GP finds an entry saying 'Glossitis, mouth gargle for 1 week' when he was about 16 years old. The young man smokes, drinks on average 36 units of alcohol per week and has a body mass index of 28.

When challenged, the young man can remember that he saw the GP as a teenager with a sore tongue, but he cannot recall exactly what happened. The GP asks the young man if he has seen this pattern on his tongue before and if this episode feels like the 'glossitis' he experienced as a teenager. The young man seems puzzled: 'I have been so worried that I might have tongue cancer. You know, I have read that smokers can develop tongue cancer and that would be awful. A workmate was recently diagnosed with tongue cancer. He was a heavy smoker. I have been so worried about it doctor'.

Examination

On examination of the tongue the GP finds red, smooth, irregular-shaped patches with a yellow elevated rim, resembling a relief map with mountain ridges (see Fig. 67.1).

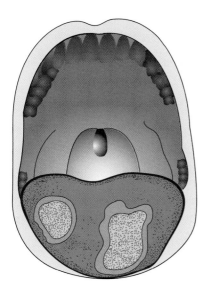

Fig. 67.1 What is the diagnosis? (illustration courtesy of Jutta Warbruck)

Questions
- What is the diagnosis?
- What tests would you initiate?
- What is the prognosis of the condition?
- What advice would you give this young man?

ANSWER

Geographic tongue (benign migratory glossitis) affects 1–2 per cent of the population and the cause is unknown. The changes to the tongue are often intermittent with long periods of remission. Exacerbating factors are spicy food, stress, smoking tobacco and cannabis. The condition is usually asymptomatic although in very troublesome cases patients complain of stinging with spicy food. The main complaint is that the tongue looks abnormal with a constantly changing appearance.

No tests are needed to confirm the diagnosis and the outlook is excellent. The condition is benign and is not known to cause any complications. Patients do not usually require any specific treatment. The young man can be reassured that the changes on his tongue are not cancer. Explaining the benign nature of his tongue condition will help the process.

The patient's worry about cancer creates a good opportunity to discuss his lifestyle and modification of his health behaviours. This young man is slightly overweight, smokes, and consumes alcohol above the recommended limit for men. Stopping smoking and eating spicy food might allow him to return to the long remission from his tongue condition that he has already experienced. Substituting healthier food, lower in energy content, will help him returning to his ideal weight. If you can convince the patient to stop smoking he is likely to reduce his alcohol intake as the two behaviours are strongly associated. It might be a good idea to make an appointment with a smoking cessation advisor there and then. Young men do not engage well with the health services and you might make it easier for him to engage by taking the first proactive steps together.

 KEY POINTS

- Patients presenting with normal variations can seem disproportionately concerned. Often they have read and/or had recent second-hand experience of a serious condition affecting the same organ. It is important to confidently identify normal variations.
- Eliciting patients' ideas and previous knowledge allows the doctor to address concerns. Recognizing the condition and communicating it to the patient, by itself, can fail to give patients adequate reassurance.
- Young men do not engage well with health-care services. Attendance at the doctor's surgery with their concerns creates a good opportunity for influencing their health behaviours.

History

A home visit has been requested for a palliative care patient. The message, taken by the receptionist from the family, is that the patient is in pain. The family is requesting an increase in the pain-killing medication and a home visit. En route the GP reflects on the situation. Six months ago the patient presented with painless obstructive jaundice. He was referred under the 2-week rule for suspected cancer. The surgeon found pancreatic cancer that was too advanced to offer surgery or any curative treatment. The patient's family has been very unhappy, saying it is all a mistake and that the NHS refused to treat him to save money. The patient deteriorated rapidly, losing weight and strength and at that time the GP thought that he had only a few days left. Then something unusual had happened. The family had asked a faith healer to attend the sick man and miraculously the jaundice disappeared and the patient felt much better. The GP had referred the patient to a gastroenterologist who put in a percutaneous endoscopic gastrostomy (PEG) tube in order to maintain his nutritional status. Initially, the patient did well, regaining his independence and attending church again. However, over the last 2 months the progression of the cancer has made itself known again and for the last 4 weeks the patient has been jaundiced once more. Pain was initially treated by oral morphine, but recently pain and nausea have increased and so the Macmillan nurses have set up a syringe driver containing anti-emetics and diamorphine.

Arriving at the house the GP is surprised to find that the whole family has gathered. The patient's wife, three children, their partners and the grandchildren are dispersed throughout the house. The patient's wife is in tears.

Examination

On examination the patient looks peaceful and comfortable. He is clearly jaundiced, but well hydrated. His pulse is calm and regular at 68 beats/minute, the blood pressure 118/74 mmHg. His respiration is irregular, oscillating between gaps and frequent deep breaths. The patient does not appear to respond, but when questioned he squeezes the GP's hand.

The oldest son approaches the GP: 'You can clearly see that my father is suffering. We want you to give my father more morphine to stop him breathing. If you don't do it, I will speed up the syringe driver and say you did it'.

Questions
- How would you respond to the son?
- How do you assess pain in an unconscious patient?
- When would the GP be justified to increase the dose of morphine?

ANSWERS

It is quite clear that the family is distressed. The GP might very well feel threatened under these circumstances and the situation needs calming down. It is important to explore the family's ideas, concerns and expectations. The setting is complicated by the past history when the family accused the NHS of a lack of treatment. They have shown a high level of support to the patient who has outlived any expectations the GP initially held for his survival. Because they have noticed his deterioration they have convened at the family home. This unusual closeness and the dying man will exert enormous stress on the family; it is understandable that the man's dying might feel protracted and unbearable for some of the family members. It is likely that the family has noticed the patient's Cheyne–Stokes respiration and they might have interpreted it as distress. The GP should explain that this pattern of breathing is normal for dying patients and that it does not cause suffering; it is the body slowly stopping functioning. The GP could explain that if the patient was in pain he would expect him to be restless and agitated and show signs of stress, with rising blood pressure and heart rate. The family may feel impotent and want to do something but not know how to help. The GP can reassure the family that being with their loved one and offering prayers or soothing words is all that he needs at this time, and that even if he appears not to respond he probably knows that those who love him are there. The GP might want to suggest that, since the man is very near the end of his life, the family may wish to summon their faith elders.

The law would not support any doctor giving an injection with the intention of killing a patient. The relative's request to increase the dose of morphine in order to stop the breathing is inappropriate. If the doctor thought that the patient was in pain it would be permissible to increase the dose of diamorphine and it would be acceptable in law that this action might hasten the patient's demise. The GP must document his actions and discussion of this visit well. He should discuss the son's inappropriate request with all the other health professionals involved in the care of this dying patient. If possible, a Macmillan or district nurse should attend the family for the last hours of the patient's life and certainly the GP should ensure that the family knows how to contact these services if needed.

 KEY POINTS

- The care of dying patients can be very stressful to the family, often reaching a climax shortly before death.
- Most families are not aware what to expect when a relative is dying and are unable to recognize normal signs and symptoms of the process.
- Patients and their families need intense support during the last days of life.

CASE 69: PALPITATIONS

History

The GP is visited by a 48-year-old woman who has noticed some palpitations over the last few weeks. She tells the GP that these can come on at any time, but particularly when she is tired and at night when she is going to sleep – she feels as if her heart is leaping in her chest. The woman owns a shoe shop locally and lives with her husband and two teenage children. Her 18-year-old daughter has recently left home and is at university in another city. Her husband is a teacher at a secondary school close by and is about to retire. They have a good relationship, although she is concerned about how he will be when he retires. Her shoe shop is very established and their children are healthy although she finds teenage children not always easy to deal with. Her 13-year-old son appears more and more disinterested in school and her 15-year-old daughter has had a few drunken episodes when she has had to be collected from parties. She misses her older daughter who has been of great support to her. She is a very sociable person and enjoys meeting up with her friends. She is generally healthy although she had an arthroscopy 2 years previously as a result of a meniscal injury. She has never smoked, exercises regularly and eats well and her body mass index (BMI) is in the normal range at 23.2. She is a great believer in herbal medicine, which she gets from the health food store. She does drink red wine regularly and her GP works out that her weekly input is about 30 units. Recently, she tells her GP that she has been feeling very tired and anxious and has lost a little weight. She had a nasty upper respiratory infection some weeks before and does not feel that she has completely recovered from this. Her periods have not been as regular as usual and when she does get them they are very heavy and last much longer than usual. She has a Nova-T intrauterine device *in situ* that has been there for the past 5 years. She has also been suffering episodes of feeling very hot and has had some diarrhoea and abdominal cramps: these remind her of the symptoms of irritable bowel syndrome that she used to suffer from. She has had a few episodes of bright red rectal bleeding that she has put down to haemorrhoids. Her father died suddenly from a myocardial infarction when he was 64 years old and her mother is still alive and well in her late 70s. Her brother has high blood pressure and high cholesterol but he is overweight and has a sedentary job.

Questions
- What does the GP need to ask about her presenting symptoms?
- What is the differential diagnosis?
- What physical examination and investigations would be particularly helpful?

The GP needs to ask more about the palpitations. It is useful to ask the patient to beat them out with her hand on the desk. How often does she have them? Are they made worse by position or exercise? Are they associated with breathlessness or chest pain? How is her exercise tolerance? Does anything else make them worse, apart from tiredness and rest? Does she drink much coffee and is she on any medications or supplements that might exacerbate them such as ginkgo biloba or ginseng? Has she had any past history of cardiac problems and has she had rheumatic fever? She tells the GP that her exercise tolerance is good although she is anxious not to do too much exercise in case it makes her palpitations worse and she is worried that she might have a heart attack. She also drinks about five strong cups of coffee a day.

The differential diagnosis includes a stress-related disorder; palpitations related to alcohol and caffeine intake; anaemia; perimenopausal symptoms; and hyperthyroidism.

The next step would include a full cardiovascular examination. Her blood pressure is slightly raised at 138/90 mmHg and her pulse is regular at 88 beats/minute. Her heart sounds are normal and there are no bruits. Abdominal examination and a rectal examination are normal, apart from a few small haemorrhoids. Because of the rectal bleeding and other symptoms the GP refers her for a colonoscopy. The GP also orders blood tests including a full blood count, thyroid function, liver function, fasting lipids and follicle-stimulating hormone (FSH). A resting electrocardiogram (ECG) and 24-hour Holter monitoring is arranged.

The blood tests come back normal with a FSH on the upper side of normal. The ECG is normal and the 24-hour reading shows a few simple ectopics. The colonoscopy is also normal. After another discussion the GP and the patient decide that her symptoms are most likely caused by early perimenopausal symptoms, anxiety and too much caffeine and alcohol. The GP suggests that the patient reduce her caffeine and alcohol intake and take up a relaxation technique. It is suggested that she and her husband go for counselling to explore his upcoming retirement and the changes that are occurring as a result of the children becoming independent.

 KEY POINTS

- Transitions, such as what is happening in this patient's life, are particular points of vulnerability.
- You might be almost certain that certain symptoms are caused by minor physical problems (for example piles), or emotional and lifestyle issues (for example life events and excess alcohol and coffee intake), but a certain level of uncertainty requires further investigation.
- The level of uncertainty at which you act is learned with experience, and if you are really not sure what to do get advice.
- Regular clinical meetings with your colleagues are valuable in sharing areas of concern and learning about how others work.

History

The on-call pager is lying on the reception desk at closing time on a Friday night. The GP responsible for Monday morning on-call has gone home without it and the receptionist asks the newly appointed GP partner to drop the pager off on his way home. The colleague's house is only one street away. There is a delay when the doorbell is rung. The young colleague is about to turn away when the door opens. His senior partner invites him in. At first the junior notices the smell, and then he is surprised to see his older colleague smoking and this is followed by an even bigger surprise when he realises that he is smoking cannabis. The senior partner offers him a smoke, but the junior partner declines and takes his leave, saying that he does not approve of drug taking.

The junior partner is upset and worried and talks to his wife. Her response comes back 'What is your problem? You told me before that he is a good doctor and a cool guy. You said that his laid-back attitude attracted you to work at his surgery. That is why you took the job. Cannabis is practically legalized in this country. Don't rock the boat'. The wife's comments do not, however, reassure him and he visits his senior partner next day for a chat. He reveals how upset he is and asks if his colleague is troubled. His senior does not display any symptoms of depression or mental illness. He admits to smoking cannabis, but he says his usage is well controlled. He likes to smoke it on Fridays after a stressful week while practising his saxophone in preparation for performing with his band in the weekend. He never smokes directly before performances as he needs to drive to the pubs where they play. The senior partner denies any alcohol problem or other illegal drug consumption. The junior asks him to stop smoking and gets told to mind his own business. On the way home the young GP is still very upset and wonders if he should inform others about his senior colleague's consumption of illegal drugs.

Questions
- What concerns might illegal drug use in a colleague raise? Did the junior colleague address them?
- Which people or organizations might be helpful in finding a solution to this problem?
- When would you involve others?

ANSWER

Most important is patient care and safety. Assessing if a fellow doctor is working safely is difficult. However, there are some indicators that could show if a colleague is in trouble:

- *Punctuality*: a colleague who displays erratic behaviour might be having a difficult time.
- *Clinical records*: good information with justifiable management plans would affirm confidence in the doctor's work.
- *Prescribing*: do the partner's prescribing patterns conform to the rest of the practice? There might be good reason if not, for example owing to a special clinical interest. Conformity is reassuring, but no guarantee of good performance.
- *Patients*: have you commonly had patients transferring to you after they have seen the other doctor and wondered why? This happens when you work with partners in a general practice, but if you see erratic management plans or ignored problems you might become suspicious.
- *The primary care team*: how do your team members find working with your colleague? Have they been let down by him? The questions can be asked without revealing the cause for concern.

It is best to address the problem with the senior colleague directly and in a timely way. Bypassing the doctor will make resolution of the problem much more difficult. If you are upset it might help you to talk with a family member or a personal friend. You must trust, however, that they realize that this information is confidential. Being new to the organization might make it difficult to understand the practice history and ways of working. A colleague might be able to help. It is important to handle the situation sensitively as the reputation of everyone is at stake.

If you do have reasonable doubts about the doctor's fitness to practise you might want to discuss your partner anonymously with your defence union before involving any other outside parties. They will help you decide if patients' care is at risk and if you need to inform others. Your clinical governance lead in your primary care trust and your local medical committee chairman are there to help. The General Medical Council is the licensing body for doctors and can investigate and remove unsafe doctors from its register.

It is your duty as a doctor to ensure patient safety. You are a partner in the surgery and you are responsible for its organization. It will not be easy to decide how covert or overt you must be in conducting your enquiries, how deeply to probe and deciding when you a satisfied enough to drop your suspicions. Nobody performs perfectly and everyone does make occasional errors of judgment. Clinical practice varies and every doctor practises medicine slightly differently. It is your decision whether to blow the whistle or not.

 KEY POINTS

- Patient safety is your highest priority.
- As a doctor you have to respond and intervene if you think a colleague is behaving unprofessionally or does not perform to an acceptable standard.
- You have a duty to look after your colleagues.

History

The appointment on your screen is for a 16-year-old girl who is currently taking the contraceptive pill. However, it is her father who comes in, to talk about her. He is obviously agitated, and angrily demands that she should be given a 'drugs test', as he thinks she is taking 'something'. Her behaviour has changed in the last year or so, from being a cheerful and outgoing schoolgirl, with plans to go to university, to a sullen, bad-tempered, disobedient teenager. She is staying out late (sometimes overnight) with her friends, lying about her whereabouts to her parents, has had a decline in her work, which has been noted by the school, is oversleeping and is untidy. You agree that the symptoms are worrying, but you cannot assess her health without seeing her. Being 16 she cannot be forced to attend, but perhaps could be persuaded to come on her own, with a parent (perhaps her mother), or with a friend. In the meantime you advise him to make contact with Adfam, a charity that offers support to families with actual or potential drug and alcohol problems; or he may prefer the National Drugs Helpline. You are careful not to discuss her medical history, particularly the Pill, even though he mentions it himself. You explain that she is now considered legally responsible for her own health care and must give her consent first. He grudgingly accepts this, and next week you see the young woman on her own.

Questions
- What questions might you ask her?
- What, if any, investigations can be suggested?
- What follow-up might be advised?

ANSWER

Establishing rapport with an unwilling patient is taxing. You will need to emphasize the confidentiality of your discussion, especially with respect to her parents. After preliminary enquiries about her general health, the Pill, etc., you might explore why her parents are concerned about her. You may wish to ask some basic health questions, including smoking, drinking and use of recreational drugs. You could specify some of the commoner drugs used by young people, such as cannabis, ecstasy, amphetamine, cocaine and heroin. If she admits to the use of any of these, you could discuss with her the reasons why she uses them. Talking about safe sex is very important.

You might observe whether she has a nasal discharge (a clue to cocaine snorting), injection marks, dilated or constricted pupils. You may feel it sensible to extend the questioning over more than one consultation to give her time to trust you. You can also talk with her about the family dynamics and school and her friendships and support.

If she consents, you could send a urine sample for toxicology drug screening, but this is usually more of forensic than clinical use. A full blood count, liver function test, hepatitis B and C screen, and *Human immunodeficiency virus* (HIV) and sexually transmitted infection testing occasionally could be considered depending on what comes out of the consultation; however, careful counselling is needed before and after these are done. The practice nurse could arrange tests.

She could be encouraged to confide in her parents, or some other trusted relative or friend, and a counsellor at her school to provide support. Your practice counsellor or a local counsellor may be able to see her. The local community mental health team or drug and alcohol service can be contacted if appropriate. She might feel uncomfortable talking about herself at the practice that her parents attend so she might choose to seek or be referred for care elsewhere. If she is internet-savvy, you could suggest some up-to-date informational internet sites appropriate for her age group. You may wish to read the Department of Health's *Drug Misuse and Dependence Guidelines.*

 KEY POINTS

- It is often difficult to know what is going on with a teenager and whether young men and women are exhibiting normal teenage behaviour or something more harmful.
- What is most important is that they have someone that they trust to talk with.
- A systemic approach looking at the whole family and social setup is always helpful.

CASE 72: RECTAL BLEEDING

History

The GP is consulted by one of her regular patients, a 46-year-old man who is unable to read or write and who has learning difficulties. The patient lives on his own in a council house where he has lived for most of his life. He was an only child, attended the local school for children with learning difficulties, and lived with his mother until she died 10 years previously, at 68 years of age, from bowel cancer. He helps a local landscape gardener for a few hours a week and is given a small wage; he also gets incapacity benefit and housing benefit. His aunt lives in a nearby town about 20 miles away and visits him about once a month. The GP has tried to get social services involved but the patient is not keen to engage with other services. The patient has not had any serious illnesses apart from minor arthritic pains for which he takes the occasional paracetamol. He is a good-natured and contented man who is well-liked in his neighbourhood. There was a time when there was concern about his vulnerability as he would invite strangers into his house but on advice from his friends and the GP this behaviour has appeared to ceased.

During the most recent consultation the patient tells the GP that he has noticed blood when his bowels move. Taking a history is difficult as he finds it hard to describe his symptoms. It appears that the patient continues to pass normal bowel motions once a day and there does not appear to be mucus with the motions. The patient has not had abdominal pains or pain when he passes a bowel motion and continues to walk and garden with as much energy as ever. He is of normal weight, and his belt buckle has been fastened at the same length for some years. He has never smoked and does not drink alcohol. His diet is simple and sensible. He tells her that he has not been eating beetroot recently. He has not had previous problems with polyps in the bowel or inflammatory bowel disease. Apart from his mother there is no family history of bowel cancer that he knows about. He did not know his father or his father's family.

Examination

The GP then takes his weight, pulse and blood pressure, which are all normal. The patient does not appear anaemic: there is no skin pallor and the conjunctivae and palmar creases are not pale. She performs a quick general examination and focuses, with the chaperone present, on an abdominal and rectal examination while carefully explaining to the patient what she is doing and why she needs to do it. There is nothing abnormal on the examination.

INVESTIGATIONS
She takes a blood test to check his haemoglobin and ferritin levels.

Questions

- How should the GP approach this consultation?
- What examinations are important?
- What should the GP do next?

ANSWER

This consultation will take extra time as taking a history and examining this patient is always slow. It is important that a proper history and examination is completed and that the patient is aware of what is going on and feels safe during the encounter. Fortunately, the patient and his doctor have known each other for several years and so there is trust between them. The GP arranges a double appointment for the next day and arranges for the practice nurse to act as a chaperone during the examination.

The GP is concerned because the patient is seldom unwell and does not generally consult for physical symptoms. She is also aware that his mother died from bowel cancer. She is not absolutely sure that the history is accurate, as she does not think that the patient completely understood all her questions and she also knows that he likes to say things to please and to prevent her from worrying about him. She talks with him about the fact that she is not sure what might be causing the bleeding and that another test, a colonoscopy that needs to be done at the hospital would make sure that all is well. She explains as well as she can what this entails. He is slightly anxious about this but agrees that she should refer him. He agrees to her letting his aunt know as he would like his aunt to accompany him to the appointment. The GP first rings the patient's aunt and explains what is going on and the aunt is keen to go with him to the hospital appointment. She then makes an urgent referral to the local hospital using the 2-week rule. The GP asks the urgent referral team to send a copy of the appointment time to her so that she can make sure that the patient and his aunt know when the appointment is, bearing in mind that the patient is unable to read.

The result of the full blood count and ferritin come back as well within normal limits. The patient is seen the next week at the colorectal clinic and an elective colonoscopy is arranged 2 weeks after that. Fortunately, there is no abnormal finding in the large bowel and the bleeding did not return. The GP is at a loss as to why the bleeding occurred. She wondered about a small anal fissure or haemorrhoid that was not visible or palpable on examination.

 KEY POINTS

- Offer a double consultation time: take your time with the patient if necessary.
- Ensure that the person consents to intervention and treatment and that they are happy for a supporter/health professional to be present during an appointment.
- People with learning difficulties need to be encouraged to speak for themselves. Talk with them in a way that they can understand and check by asking them to tell you in their own words what they think is going on.

History

A 23-year-old nursery worker has been sent home from work and advised to see her doctor. The previous day she had developed a sore throat and watering eyes and had felt hot and cold. The morning of her GP visit her eyes felt sticky and gritty when she awoke and when she looked into the mirror she noticed that the whites of her eyes seemed red and her eye lids looked swollen. Her neck was hurting and her throat was still slightly sore. In the past few days the nursery had send home several children with conjunctivitis. The nursery policy is not to allow children back until 48 hours after eye treatment has been initiated.

Examination

On examination the GP notices lateral inflammation of the conjunctivae and normal corneae bilaterally. Her throat is slightly reddened and there are multiple tender swollen lymph nodes in the pre-auricular region and down her neck. She denies any blurred or impaired vision. Her temperature is 37.6°C.

The GP tell his patient that the cause of sore throat and red eyes is likely to be viral. He advises her to wash her hands regularly and use a separate towel to lessen the risk of transmitting her illness to anyone else. He tells her that she is fit to return to work once she feels better and that she requires no specific treatment.

The nursery nurse seems uncomfortable: 'I don't understand. I thought that conjunctivitis is dangerous and can cause blindness. We require our children to be treated with antibiotic eye drops before they can return. Why aren't you giving me any treatment, doctor?'

Questions
- What are the most likely causative agents for this patient's conjunctivitis?
- Should patients with conjunctivitis be excluded from nursery?
- What treatments could the GP offer to his patient?
- Is the patient's sight in danger?

ANSWER

There appears to be an outbreak of pharyngoconjunctival fever (conjunctivitis associated with upper respiratory tract infection) at the nursery. This condition is usually caused by adenoviral infection. Viral conjunctivitis is usually bilateral, although it can be asymmetrical. Patients might suffer from mild photophobia when the cornea is affected. Viral conjunctivitis is spread by droplet infection and there is an increased risk of spread in any situation where people are in regular close contact as in the nursery. The risk of spread can be reduced by careful hand-washing and rigorous use of separate towels. The disease is mild and rapidly self-limiting but may occasionally be severe and disabling. The table below contrasts the three most common causes of an acutely painful red eye.

Conjunctivitis is not on the list of conditions from the Department of Health or Health Protection Agency where absence from school until the child is well is recommended. However, they suggest that parents may choose to keep their children off school until they feel better and that, occasionally, if there is an outbreak in a nursery or school, parents might be asked to keep their children at home until the infection is cleared but that this is not usually required. No treatment is a common option for mild or moderate infections and without treatment most cases of infective conjunctivitis clear on their own within 1–2 weeks, and often within 2–5 days. Bathing the eyes with cool clean water may be soothing and lubricant eye drops may reduce eye discomfort. These are available over the counter, as well as on prescription.

The nursery worker's fear of losing her eye-sight is not, in her case, founded on medical evidence. However, blindness following infection of the conjunctivae can be caused by herpes or chlamydial infection, the latter usually presenting as a severe form of conjunctivitis with generalized hyperaemia and profuse mucopurulent discharge. In the economically underdeveloped world ocular serovars of *Chlamydia trachomatis*, or trachoma, are the most common infectious cause of blindness.

 KEY POINTS

- Patients sometimes have an understanding of common diseases that conflict with the views of health professionals.
- Institutions might have policies excluding children from nursery or school that are not based on recommendations from the Department of Health or the Health Protection Agency.

Table 73.1

Condition	Degree of pain	Photophobia	Discharge	Redness	Cornea	Pupil	Intraocular pressure
Acute conjunctivitis	Roughness on lid movements	Slight	Clear or purulent	Generalized redness of the conjunctiva	Normal	Normal	Normal
Acute iritis	Dull ache within the eye	Severe	Slight reflex watering	Circum-corneal redness	Deposits on lower surface	May be small	Normal
Acute glaucoma	Severely painful eye	Moderate	Slight reflex watering	Circum-corneal duskiness	Haze over the anterior surface	Fixed dilated, oval	Raised

History

A 68-year-old Afro-Caribbean man attends the surgery for a routine appointment. He holds a letter from the surgery asking him to return for a follow-up appointment because of abnormalities found in his blood test: 'I have been so worried doctor. When I got this letter I phoned up and asked the receptionist about the results. She talked with the nurse who said that my kidney function tests are abnormal and that I have got Stage 3 Chronic Kidney Disease. My mother had to have dialysis for kidney disease and she died from it so quickly'. The GP checks the history. 'I can see that we arranged a blood test as part of routine monitoring of your blood pressure treatment. According to my records your blood pressure has been well controlled by your ramipril tablets over the last year. All your blood pressure readings have been below the target value of 135/80mmHg'. Checking the prescription record he finds that the patient had ordered and collected his prescription for ramipril regularly at 8-weekly intervals. 'My records show that your high blood pressure was detected 15 years ago. I can't find any other recorded past medical problems. Is that correct? Good. My records also show that you have a family history of diabetes. It says your mother suffered from it. Did she have high blood pressure as well? I can't find any abnormal results looking through your previous blood tests. Your kidney function has always been within normal limits. However, the specialists have developed a new way of combining your age, sex and creatinine to estimate your kidney function called the estimated glomerular filtration rate, or eGFR. Your result came back as 53. Values below 60 put you at Stage 3 Chronic Kidney Disease (CKD). The guidelines suggest that patients in Stages 3–5 of the disease should be referred to a kidney specialist. Would this be OK with you?'

Questions
- How would you interpret this patient's eGFR?
- How would you further assess patients with Stage 3 CKD?
- For what other disease is Stage 3 CKD a good risk indicator?

ANSWER

The GP failed to adjust the eGFR for black patients. The patient's true eGFR is therefore 53 × 1.21 or 64.13 mL/minute. A patient's predicted eGFR is also dependent on the patient age, reducing by about 10 mL per decade.

!							
Age	40	50	60	70	80	90	100
eGFR	100	90	80	70	60	50	40

The patient's eGFR is close to the value expected for his age and ethnicity. In addition the GP also failed to understand that CKD cannot be diagnosed on the basis of eGFR alone. There should also be other evidence of kidney disease such as proteinuria, haematuria, evidence of structurally abnormal kidneys or genetic diagnosis of kidney disease. The blood test could be repeated after a week to confirm the result. Deteriorating renal function would necessitate referral to the renal team.

If the doctor's initial assessment had been correct and the patient had Stage 3 CKD a more detailed assessment would be required but usually community care is appropriate as long as kidney function is stable. Asking questions such as is the patient well and is there a history of significant associated disease would be important. Examination for bladder enlargement would indicate imaging if obstruction is suspected and is also indicated if there is severe hypertension or declining GFR. A medication review would reveal any potentially nephrotoxic drugs, or drugs that need dose alterations when the GFR reduces. Additional blood tests, including those for serum electrolytes, serum calcium, serum phosphate, haemoglobin level, serum cholesterol and parathyroid hormone would be required. Hypercalcaemia may cause acute renal impairment or deterioration. The GP should carry out a dipstick for blood and protein, and quantify positive proteinuria by a protein–creatinine ratio. A cardiovascular assessment, including blood pressure and peripheral circulation, is important and severe hypertension despite multiple agents may be an indication for referral. The risk of cardiovascular events and death is substantially increased for all stages of CKD and on average is higher than the risk of needing dialysis or a renal transplant. Long-term monitoring and review is required.

In this situation there was no other evidence of kidney disease and so the patient was not finally diagnosed with CKD. The GP had to explain this to him, much to the relief of the patient who had had a nasty shock. Being told that they have chronic kidney disease can have a profound effect on patients, and on their health beliefs and self-efficacy. Doctors should take care to make the correct diagnosis and (if necessary) in giving bad news.

KEY POINTS

- Abnormal blood tests are not synonymous with disease.
- Take care to make the correct diagnosis.
- Be aware of the impact of giving bad news to patients.

History

The next patient is a 27-year-old man, who limps into the consulting room on two crutches, with his left leg in a below-knee plaster, and sutures on his forehead. He says that 3 weeks ago he accidentally drove into a tree, and woke to find himself in hospital. The discharge letter he gives you reveals that he suffered a head injury with loss of consciousness, and a compound fracture of his tibia/fibula. He was in the intensive therapy unit for some days, under neurological assessment, and has had an internal fixation of his fracture. A magnetic resonance imaging (MRI) scan of the head showed no major damage. Apart from some pain-killers, and a course of antibiotics, he is on no medication. He is obviously downcast and he asks for a certificate for work.

While writing this, you ask him about the accident: was anyone else hurt: 'No'. How badly damaged was the car: 'A write-off'. Were the police involved: 'Yes'. In fact, he was breathalysed and will be appearing in court on a charge of drunk driving. This is not the first time, and he is facing a driving ban, which would result in him losing his job as a van driver. He already has problems at home, as he is separated from his partner, and was in fact returning from a visit to see his two young sons for the first time since a court order banning him was lifted. As a result of the accident, he may also lose this access privilege too.

Questions
- What further questions would be helpful to ask now?
- To whom could you refer him for further help?
- What medication might you be able to offer him?

ANSWER

First, is he suffering any late sequelae from the head injury: headaches, blurred or double vision, or seizures? As he is not, no urgent referral back to the neurologist seems indicated. Next, you ask about his drinking habits. It appears he is accustomed to drink at least 50 units of alcohol a week, and thinks this is nothing unusual. He admits to disturbed sleep even before the accident, and hints that the break-up of his relationship was caused in some part by his drinking. Using the CAGE tool, he scores 3 out of a possible 4 points:

- he has not seriously thought about *Cutting down*;
- he has been *Annoyed* by criticism;
- he now feels *Guilty*;
- he does take a morning *Eye-opener* drink to relieve hangover.

This tool identifies dependent drinkers, focusing on lifetime drinking habits as with this man, with two positive answers considered a positive result. Other alcohol tools that are used at present in primary care include the FAST screening tool that identifies hazardous drinking, including binge drinking, and the AUDIT or a shortened AUDIT questionnaire that can be used if the FAST tool picks up possible hazardous drinking (you can find the details of these screening tools on the internet). AUDIT focuses more carefully on the preliminary signs of hazardous and harmful drinking and identifying mild dependence.

The patient is now amenable to advice about his drinking problem. After exploring his options (total abstinence, drinking less than 21 units/week, cutting back 'a bit' or carrying on unchanged) you can suggest that he seeks more formal advice from local alcohol services and give him the contact details. Depending on his motivation he will be offered 'detox' and rehabilitation. During detox sedatives will be required to prevent the symptoms of uncomplicated alcohol withdrawal, delirium tremens and withdrawal seizures, and vitamins will be given (including thiamine) to prevent the development of Wernicke's encephalopathy. You advise him not to reduce his intake until he gets specialist advice and assistance in order to avoid serious physical and emotional sequelae. In the meantime, you start him on some vitamin B complex, thiamine and vitamin C tablets as his alcohol intake is high, and chronic, and his diet poor.

His consultation has now lasted half-an-hour, instead of the allotted 10 minutes. Although your schedule is shot to pieces, you hope that your concern for his welfare, and a non-judgmental attitude, will encourage him to return for follow-up, and you ask him to come back in 2 weeks, booking a double appointment.

 KEY POINTS

- It has been estimated that, in the UK, more than 9 out of 10 people drink alcohol; about 1 in 3 men and 1 in 6 women have some sort of health problem caused by alcohol; around 1 in 15 men and 1 in 50 women are physically dependent on alcohol.
- Problems with alcohol are common and the cost in physical, psychological, social and economic terms substantial: screen all adult patients.
- GPs have a responsibility to inform patients of the harmful effects of alcohol and provide advice on alcohol treatment and rehabilitation services; the responsibility for seeking help lies with the patient.

CASE 76: SELF-HARM

History

One of your patients is a 63-year-old woman with a long history of hypertension. You are aware that her mother died from the complications of Huntington's disease and that her brother, who is 2 years older than she, also suffers from Huntington's disease. Her brother is married and has a very supportive wife and three children in their 20s. He learned of his diagnosis 10 years previously when he developed slight uncontrollable movements, increasing clumsiness and depression. The patient lives alone and has never married because of her fear of passing on Huntington's disease to any children. She was also heavily involved in caring for her mother until she died 20 years ago and had no time to develop relationships. She has not been tested as she prefers not to know whether or not she carries the gene. She has worked as a carer for the local authority and retired 3 years previously as she found the work too physically demanding.

You have not seen her for a few months when you get a phone call from your local hospital to say that she has recently been seen in the Accident and Emergency Department with a suicide attempt. She makes an appointment to see you and you find out that recently she has been drinking heavily and feeling very low and isolated. She had been too ashamed to see you and eventually felt so bad that she drank a bottle of whisky and took a number of co-dydramol tablets. Luckily she had second thoughts and rang her sister-in-law to tell her of her action; she called an ambulance and treatment was initiated before any lasting damage was done. A number of consultations follow at weekly intervals as you explore with her the situation and reasons for her unhappiness. You discover that she is very concerned that she may have Huntington's disease as one of her mother's and brother's symptoms was depression. She has had a problem with alcohol in the past and is very aware that she drinks more heavily when she is feeling low. She is also very worried about her brother as he appears to be getting sicker and more dependent on his family.

Questions
- What is the role of the GP in this kind of scenario?
- What is Huntington's disease?
- What are the common genetic disorders we deal with in general practice?

ANSWER

For the GP this is a situation where many skills are being asked for. The patient has a pre-existing physical disorder – hypertension – which needs ongoing care. The GP also needs to care for this patient's psychological and emotional well-being very carefully as the patient is at risk of further suicide attempts. The patient's alcohol problem needs to be addressed. The doctor also needs to support the patient to come to a decision about whether she would now want DNA testing for possible Huntington's disease.

Huntington's disease is a single gene disorder caused by a malfunctioning gene on chromosome 4. It is an autosomal dominant disease and is a progressive neurodegenerative disorder. If one parent has the disorder their children will have a 50 per cent chance of having the faulty gene and all people who have this gene will develop the disease at some stage. The condition affects about 1 in 15000 people across much of the world and equally affects men and women. The early symptoms vary but can include memory loss or confusion, changes in personality and mood and slight uncontrolled muscle movements. As the disease progresses these symptoms become more severe and it is invariably fatal. The early symptoms usually start between 30 and 50 years of age but it can start at any age and symptoms can differ from person to person. A genetics test is available.

General practitioners, with their role in the long-term care of patients and their families, are ideally placed to take an active role in the diagnosis and treatment of genetic disorders. Common activities in this arena include preconception counselling and prenatal testing for genetic disorders such as Down's syndrome, pre-symptomatic DNA testing in families where there is a genetic disorder, such as familial adenomatous polyposis, haemochromatosis, Huntington's disease or specific cancer genes such as *BRCA1* or *BRCA2* (a rare cause of ovarian or breast cancer) and community DNA screening for populations at risk of such diseases as sickle cell or thalassaemia.

 KEY POINTS

- Genetic disorders need to be seen in the context of a person's life and community.
- Huntington's disease, in its final phase, is a serious and debilitating disease and this genetic disorder requires careful support and monitoring from the time of diagnosis.
- What is a genetic 'disorder' for some may be regarded simply as a genetic 'difference' for others. Take care not to assume anything when talking with patients and families.

CASE 77: SEXUAL ABUSE

History

A girl of 13 years of age sees her GP accompanied by her mother. They both appear anxious and the girl is very withdrawn. She is finding it hard to explain why she has consulted the GP so her mother tells what has happened. She tells you, that, during a recent holiday to the seaside, her daughter had developed mild vaginitis that required a trip to the doctor. After this consultation the girl disclosed to her mother that she had been recently sexually abused by a neighbour. The girl lives with her mother and her younger sister of 11 years of age. They live in a council house not far from the surgery and both girls go to the local school. The mother is a good and caring mother, although life is not easy as she has very little money and has not had a good education. She works long hours as a hospital cleaner, sometimes not being at home when the girls get back from school. The girl's father does not have contact with them, having left when the youngest was aged 3 years, and is now living with his second wife and their young family in a town 200 miles away. The two girls have generally had good health apart from eczema and asthma, both are somewhat overweight and the eldest (this patient) does have mild learning difficulties and has had input from an educational psychologist.

Questions
- What does the GP do now?
- What services are available for this family's care?

ANSWER

The GP has a responsibility to provide care and protection to the young girl and her sister. An urgent referral needs to be made to the child protection services as well as ensuring that the girl's physical symptoms have been or will be fully investigated and treated as necessary. First, it is helpful to gather more information from the girl and her mother. The girl may feel better talking with you alone or with her mother present and you can ask her what she prefers and negotiate this with her and her mother. It would be helpful to know a little more about the abuse, for example who the perpetrator is, what has happened, how often it has happened and over how long it has been taking place. The GP needs to find out about the consultation with the doctor at the seaside resort and whether or not investigations had taken place at this time. The GP may well want to contact this doctor and find out more about that consultation. The GP does not examine the girl, leaving this to a doctor who has the expertise and experience. She may also be suffering from a sexually transmitted disease, or may even be pregnant. Her younger sister may also be at risk of abuse. The GP talks with the mother and the child about the necessity to involve social services and why this is important. In this case, the mother and the daughter agree that referral is important. The GP contacts the local social services duty manager by phone and follows this up immediately with a written referral. Clear notes are made in the child's medical record.

The main services that need to know about this situation are social services and the police. A medical practitioner with special training will also be involved and will investigate the physical symptoms.

 KEY POINTS

- The GP's chief responsibility is to the well-being of the child or children concerned.
- It is essential to keep clear, accurate, comprehensive and contemporaneous notes.
- Concerns need to be reported promptly to social services or the police.
- The GP should only give information to those who need to know.

CASE 78: SEXUAL ABUSE

History

The GP is seeing a family of mother and two daughters aged 13 and 11 years where sexual abuse has been disclosed by the 13-year-old (see Case 77). The mother reported this to the GP and the situation has been referred to the local child protection services. Over recent weeks the child protection team, involving social services, child health services, the police, education services and the GP, have made a full investigation. It has emerged that a 19-year-old neighbour of the family had sexually abused the 13-year-old on one occasion. It does not appear that the 11-year-old sister has been abused. This has led to the 19-year-old being held on bail, awaiting a court appearance. It is felt that he is not safe to be at large in the community and it also appears that he had regularly sexually abused another young girl in the community and that this had not previously come to light. The 13-year-old originally went to the doctor because of mild vaginitis and this has been shown to be a mild *Candida* infection that has cleared with treatment. Investigations have revealed no sexually transmitted disease and she is not pregnant. She is now back at school. The child protection services have decided that the children are safe in their own home with extra support and regular follow-up. Because of their mother needing to work they are often home alone in the afternoons when they get back from school. Although the law does not set a minimum age at which children can be left alone it is evident that these two girls are vulnerable, especially since the 13-year-old has mild learning difficulties. Her mother is so distressed about what has happened that she has been unable to work and is on sick leave. They are having family counselling and support from social and education services.

The mother has made an appointment to see the GP.

Questions
- How should the GP handle this consultation?
- What interventions could support the mother and her family?

ANSWER

The GP is there to be of support to the mother; however, the prime responsibility of the GP is the safety of the two daughters. Part of the consultation will be to assess the mental and physical health of the mother and her continued ability to care for her children. The mother reports that she is very angry and saddened by what has happened and feels very responsible for what transpired. She has gone through agony thinking that her children may have been taken away from her. The GP reiterates how important it was that she responded so quickly and properly when she had heard from her daughter what had happened. She tells the doctor that her 13-year-old has, of course, been very disturbed by what has happened but that she seems to have returned to some kind of normality relatively quickly. The 11-year-old has been very carefully treated throughout the whole episode and appears almost untouched by it. The mother is now eating and sleeping better than she was before but does not feel strong enough to return to work. She is worried that she is now being overprotective of her children, dropping them at school in the morning, picking them up after school and not allowing them to go outside on their own. The GP explains to her that this is to be expected and that her extreme fear may take some time to pass: she is having regular counselling from victim support to help her to adjust. She is more concerned about the future and who will look after her children when she returns to work.

The GP talks with her about the possibilities. One idea is that she move to Ireland to live near her sister who has similar-aged children. They can share child-care responsibilities and support each other to work. In some ways this situation has highlighted what she has been feeling for a long time – that she has been struggling with little support and little money. She worries for her children and does need to find a more supportive living situation. She does not have family close by and her friends are all in similar situations although a few have offered to help share the child-care. There are real possibilities here, although at present she does not trust anyone apart from her family with the safety of her children. The GP extends her sickness certificate for another month and asks her to return in 3 weeks for further discussion.

 KEY POINTS

- This situation will take time to come to some resolution and the GP needs to give it the space to do so.
- The safety and well-being of the children must continue to be paramount.
- The GP needs to continue to stay in touch with the child protection team.

History

An 18-year-old young woman returns to see her GP requesting a renewal of her sick note. She had missed her last two appointments at the surgery, 1 and 2 weeks previously. Six weeks before this consultation she had been seen by a fellow GP who wrote in her notes: 'Never worked in her life, fit to work which will benefit her condition'.

The GP reviews the records. He had seen the patient for the first time 10 months previously when she was brought in by her aunt who reported that her mood was very low. It emerged that her boyfriend had left her 2 months beforehand and that she had found it difficult to cope, withdrawing from all social activities. She lived at home with her parents but they were out most of the time and not much involved in her care. During the first interview it was the aunt who did all the talking, the young woman remaining silent. The aunt seemed to be genuinely worried about the girl: 'I can't be with her all the time and she is not right'.

At the first consultation the young woman had been issued with a sickness certificate at that point for 2 months. Since then she had attended various GPs in the practice and had been issued with ongoing certificates. She had been referred to the practice-based psychologist who had seen her for an assessment, diagnosed mild depression and offered therapy, but the girl failed to attend further sessions and was subsequently discharged back to the GP.

Examination

On examination the girl is well-groomed, quiet with her gaze lowered. Her answers to questions on her well-being are monosyllabic. She denies suicidal intent or plans to harm herself. Enquiries on her daily activities are unfruitful as she does not engage in any conversation. She denies alcohol or drug abuse. Running out of options the GP asks the patient if anything has been helpful and she answers in the negative. Asking what might help, in her opinion, to get better gets a 'don't know' answer. Challenged about why she thought that she was unable to work she says that she is depressed and does not want to go out of the house. She is not willing to accept any therapy. The GP challenges the patient again saying that a fellow GP had voiced the opinion that she was fit to work, but the patient insists that she needs the sick note in order to claim her benefits. Could the GP please backdate the note allowing her claim money for all the time that she has been unable to work?

Questions
- Confronted with this situation, how do you think the GP feels?
- Do you think that the GP should give the young woman a sick note?

ANSWER

The GP is likely to feel helpless and overwhelmed. The patient has failed to benefit from any of the numerous therapeutic attempts the surgery has offered. There a conflict between the patient's request for a sick note and the documented opinion from one of the GP's colleagues that she is fit to work.

Patients who provoke negative emotional responses in doctors have been termed 'heart-sink patients'. The young woman appears to have a child-like attitude in failing to engage with any therapeutic relationship with health-care professionals. Seeing the name of the patient, the GP may have a feeling of impending doom, knowing that no matter how much time and empathy is poured into the consultation, the outcome is unlikely to change the patient's health status. With the way that the consultation has gone the GP might feel sad and a failure, or angry and upset about the girl's lack of response, or even experience all these emotions at once. The doctor will also be anxious not to miss signs of suicidal intend or impending self-harming behaviours. It is likely that the GP will be trying to avoid direct conflict with the patient.

Sick certification by doctors allows patients to take on the sick role excusing them from having to undertake certain expectations and responsibilities. In return, patients are obliged to show that they are trying to get better, regaining their health in order to return to normal duties or roles. Discussing this with the patient with another referral to mental health services might be in order.

Society expects doctors to use their powers in legitimizing illness justly and wisely. It is difficult to measure a person's fitness to work and is the field of occupational health specialists. Most GPs will follow the patients' own perceptions of fitness to work, if it seems reasonable. Doctors might feel they are in conflict over a patient's perception of fitness to work and their duty towards society. The benefit system gives GPs the opportunity to report that they have given a sick note under duress.

In this case the GP completes an RM7 form and sends it to the manager of the local Department for Work and Pensions office and asks for an independent assessment of the patient's ongoing incapacity to work. The RM7 form is found at the back of the Med 3 or Med 4 pads. It does not ask for any clinical information.

 KEY POINTS

- Doctors may experience powerful emotions dealing with patients and some patient groups are more likely to evoke 'heart-sink' feelings.
- The role of patient sickness is a complicated social construct and it is important that doctors are aware of the consequences of legitimizing patients' illnesses.
- It is sometimes hard to tell whether there is an underlying mental health problem or not and, in this situation, seeking a second opinion is important.

History

An 18-month-old infant is brought to his GP by his mother. He presents with depigmentation on his chest and abdomen. The white areas have become more noticeable over the summer. He was seen 4 months previously with a similar rash and a diagnosis of ringworm was made. He was treated with miconazole cream, but his mother soon ran out of the cream and did not get a repeat prescription. The mother is worried about psoriasis as the child's father suffers from this condition. There is no other family history of skin disease and the infant is otherwise healthy. He and his family are well known by the practice. The infant lives with his mother in a one-bedroom council flat. He has no siblings and his father does not live with them but visits regularly, has a close relationship with him and is a good support to his mother. He does not go to stay at his father's flat and is not in nursery although he does regularly visit the local '1 o'clock' club with his mother. His maternal grandparents enjoy caring for him and this also gives his parents a break.

Examination

On examination the child has large irregularly shaped, asymmetrical, slightly scaly patches of depigmentation on his chest and abdomen and multiple bruises on his shins. He appears happy and well-adjusted if a little shy. He is walking and getting into everything. He can say a few words.

Questions
- What is the diagnosis?
- Are any further investigations are needed?
- What advice do you give mother?

ANSWER

The diagnosis is pityriasis versicolor. It is caused by a commensal yeast, *Pityrosporum obiculare*. Some people seem to be more prone to develop this skin infection than others and hot, sunny and humid weather seem to be a common trigger. The child was seen at an early stage and only partially treated. The untreated infected areas have not tanned in the sun and so have become more obvious.

> The differential diagnosis includes vitiligo but this presents as white completely depigmented patches of otherwise normal skin with the distribution of patches usually symmetrical.

If the diagnosis is in doubt, skin scrapings can be taken. The bruises on the shin are normal for an active toddler of this age. We might think of possible abuse but the bruising is confined to his shins, the infant has a good relationship with his mother and father and, apart from his grandparents, no-one else is involved in his care. All these mitigate against the possibility.

The application of cream to large areas of skin is difficult. Treatment for 5 days with an antifungal shampoo (ketoconazole 2 per cent) is easier and effective. Recurrence of the infection can be prevented by continuing the treatment once weekly for the next 6 months. The condition is regarded as non-infectious. The parents need to be aware that the depigmentation will stay after the treatment until a new suntan is achieved. This often takes 2–6 months.

KEY POINTS

- It is important to take a history of dermatological complaints. Reported facts might be skewed, but often still illuminate the problem (history of ringworm treatment).
- Patients need to be given information allowing them to judge the success of treatments and how long signs might persist, even after successful therapy.
- Always consider the possibility of abuse when seeing patients with bruises or injuries and look out for signs. However, not all bruises are sign of non-accidental injury.
- Look on the internet for images of pityriasis versicolor. Good websites are those of the British Association of Dermatologists, American Academy of Dermatology, New Zealand Dermatological Society, and DermAtlas.

CASE 81: SKIN RASH

History

A mother brings in her 5-year-old twins. She is worried that they might have developed chickenpox for the third time: 'I thought you can get them only once'. She reports that one boy had the spots first, developing spots on his arms, then his legs and finally on his trunk. The other boy has developed a lesser number of spots, mainly affecting his arms. Mother denies any general upset in the children, with no fever, loss of energy or appetite.

The GP reviews the records and finds one confirmed episode of chickenpox 18 months ago. The entry in the notes says: 'Chickenpox rash, spots developing in crops, mild febrile illness, for calamine lotion and paracetamol'. Mother reports that she did not attend for the second episode of chickenpox as the family was abroad at the time and she already knew what to do. The GP notices that the more badly affected twin has a history of eczema needing regular emollient therapy.

Examination

Examination of the more badly affected twin shows skin-coloured papules concentrated on the inside of his forearms and elbow creases, in both axillae and on the flexor side of his knees, with a few single papules on the front of his chest and abdomen. The papules are up to 5 mm in size and some have a small central dimple.

Questions

- What is the diagnosis?
- How do you explain the distribution on the worse-affected twin?
- How would you treat this condition?

ANSWER

The diagnosis is molluscum contagiosum, a common skin condition caused by a pox-virus. The 1–5 mm papules with a central punctum are typical. When the papule gets squeezed a white cheesy substance containing the live virus is released through the punctum. The condition is harmless: it can cause minor local irritation but does not cause generalized illness in patients. It is passed on by direct skin-to-skin contact and children often spread the condition by scratching open a papule and spreading the infected contents. Each lesion lasts about 6–12 weeks and crops of papules tend to erupt over 12–18 months. Sufferers develop a lasting immunity to the virus.

Textbooks and common wisdom often tell us that you can get chickenpox only once. However, studies of children with a suspected second episode of chickenpox have shown that these patients have developed an insufficient immune response after the first infection. It appears that a minority of children can develop more than one episode of chickenpox infection. The child might therefore have had a second bout of chickenpox; however, this rash is not chickenpox.

The worse-affected twin suffers with eczema. Children with atopic dermatitis often experience worse eruptions of this disease. The sites of the lesions can be explained by scratching of the typically worst-affected eczematous areas in the flexor areas of large joints.

First-line management of this condition is watchful waiting as the cure for children can be worse than the condition. An area of redness around a lesion suggests an immune response and clearance.

The lesions usually disappear within 18 months and no restriction from school or swimming pools is necessary. If treatment is considered necessary, expressing the white core infected material after bathing, a few at a time with careful disposal of the expressed material or repeated cryotherapy are options.

 KEY POINTS

- Sometimes research refutes common wisdom and textbook knowledge.
- It is best to question a patient's self-made diagnoses, especially when they already question it themselves.
- Look for pictures of molluscum contagiosum on the internet if you are not sure what these lesions look like. Good websites are those of the British Association of Dermatologists, American Academy of Dermatology, New Zealand Dermatological Society, and DermAtlas.

CASE 82: SKIN RASH

History

A 6-year-old boy is brought to surgery by his mother. He was seen 1 week previously, generally well but for an acute generalized rash. The doctor made a diagnosis of an acute allergic rash although no trigger was found and the boy was treated with an anti-histamine. His mother brings him back today because he has not improved. He lives with his parents and one older brother and they have a pet dog that they have had for 5 years. It is winter and, because the weather has been unseasonably warm, the boy has recently spent lots of time in the garden playing football with his brother and his father. He does not suffer from hay fever, asthma or eczema. His mother tells the GP that he has not eaten anything out of the ordinary and that she has not recently changed soaps or washing powder. No other family members or friends have similar rashes and the boy has had no other symptoms. The rash is slightly itchy.

Examination

On examination the boy is well and apyrexial. He has a generalized rash covering his trunk and, to a lesser degree, his limbs. The rash consists of 1–3 cm oval patches, some showing mild scaling on the inner side of its borders. The patches seem to form lines following the skin creases. On questioning, his mother does remember that one patch erupted on his chest 5 days before the rash generalized.

Questions
- What is the diagnosis?
- What advice do you give to the mother?

ANSWER

The diagnosis is pityriasis rosea, a skin condition commonly seen in general practice. The patches following the skin creases, the herald patch and the scaling on the inside of the border of some of the patches in a well child make the diagnosis certain. Parents might forget to tell the doctor about the herald patch or it might go unnoticed. The cause is unknown but because the illness occurs in clusters and is most common in winter it is thought that it might be of viral origin, although no specific virus has been identified. The acute onset caught the first doctor, who diagnosed the allergic rash, off guard. The rash looks alarming and mother needs strong reassurance. It is important to tell her that the disease is of a benign nature, and that the rash can take up to 8 weeks to fade away, occasionally longer. The risk of passing it on to anyone else is very low. No treatment is needed other than symptomatic treatment such as calamine lotion prescribed for the occasional patient who suffers with itchiness. A second attack is very unlikely.

 KEY POINTS

- Pityriaisis rosea is a disease that is commonly misdiagnosed. The history of a herald patch and the scaling on the lesions are pathognomonic.
- Rashes, even benign ones, cause a great deal of anxiety to patients and their parents. Providing a diagnosis gives them the reassurance they seek.
- Look for pictures of pityriasis rosea on the internet if you are not sure what this rash looks like. Good websites are those of the British Association of Dermatologists, American Academy of Dermatology, New Zealand Dermatological Society, and DermAtlas.

History

An 8-year-old boy is brought after school to his GP by his mother. He has been slightly unwell for the last 3 days complaining of intermittent mild headaches, slightly achy limbs and a slight fever. He has had no vomiting or diarrhoea. Today at school he has developed a bright red rash on both cheeks. His teacher had noticed his red cheeks but had not thought it serious enough to contact his mother. About 2 weeks ago he had been in contact with a family friend with similar symptoms. He has had chickenpox and is up to date with all his immunizations. Mother is concerned that the boy will be very upset if he cannot attend school as he has a star role in a school play in a few days time and is in the midst of rehearsals. He has one younger sister who has not been unwell and his family are all healthy and rarely come to the doctor except for immunizations and health checks.

Examination

On examination he has a bright red rash on both cheeks, he is alert and in no pain and is feeling quite well although a little tired. His temperature is 37.6°C. His throat and ears are normal, he has no other rash, chest and abdominal examinations are normal and there is no neck stiffness.

Question

- What is the diagnosis?
- Are there any complications associated with the condition?
- What advice do you give to the mother?

ANSWER

The diagnosis is slapped cheek disease (fifth disease, erythema infectiosum) which is caused by parvovirus B19. It is contagious for 4–20 days before the rash appears. Typically, children aged 4–12 years contact the disease. A faint rash can appear on the trunk and limbs. Usually the rash comes and disappears within a few days, but occasionally it fades and returns for up to 4 weeks. Twenty to thirty per cent of those acutely infected remain asymptomatic. You might think of the possibility of meningitis but there are no signs to suggest this, in particular no high fever, cold hands and feet, severe leg pain, very pale or mottled skin, severe headache, photophobia, neck stiffness, nausea and vomiting, drowsiness or other skin rash, and the rash is blanching.

Slapped cheek disease can trigger an aplastic anaemia in children with sickle cell disease, β-thalassaemia and spherocytosis. The disease can also trigger a miscarriage or cause fetal abnormalities in non-immune pregnant women, especially before the 20th week of gestation.

The mother should be advised that the boy be allowed to return to school when he seems fit to go. If the sibling is infected she might show symptoms 4–20 days after first contact with the disease. The boy should be kept away from individuals who might be harmed by the virus, although by the time the rash appears it is normally no longer infectious. These guidelines are outlined on the Health Protection Agency website and can be shown to the mother if she is unsure about the wisdom of your advice.

 KEY POINTS

- Infectious diseases in children are common. By the time they see the doctor infectivity has often passed.
- Parents are concerned to fulfil their public duty in containing infectious diseases and schools and nurseries often have overcautious protocols not necessarily based on Department of Health or Health Protection Agency guidelines.
- Make sure you have a resource handy for looking up incubation times and infectivity of common diseases. The Health Protection Agency website is a useful reference point.
- Look for pictures of slapped cheek disease on the internet if you are not sure what this rash looks like. Good websites are those of the British Association of Dermatologists, American Academy of Dermatology, New Zealand Dermatological Society, and DermAtlas.

CASE 84: SKIN RASH

History

A 29-year-old builder presents to his GP with a week-long history of sores on his penis. The sores developed after sexual intercourse with his ex-wife when his foreskin ripped and bled. He noticed redness and itching on his penis and, on the next day, the skin on these areas became wet. He then started to develop headaches, muscle pains, general malaise and feeling hot with intermittent shivers. The patient also reports irritation in the urethra on and after micturition. He has not noticed any penile discharge. When the pain increased he attended the Accident and Emergency Department of his local hospital where the doctor prescribed flucloxacillin. A small abscess on his shoulder had improved on the antibiotics but the penile sores persisted.

The patient and his ex-wife had divorced 3 years previously and since their split had formed a common household with their daughter. The mother had been living with another man for 2 years, while the patient had been sexually abstinent. They had got back together only recently and had not used condoms or any contraception as a child would be a welcome outcome. The couple engaged in oral and penetrative vaginal sex but since the development of symptoms the couple had not engaged in sexual intercourse. The patient told the GP that he had not had any sexually transmitted infection diagnosed or treated in the past. His ex-wife denied any symptoms of infection. His past medical history reveals a road traffic accident 1 year ago, herpes labialis (cold sore) 3 years ago, epididymitis 4 years ago, cellulitis of his leg 10 years ago and a perforated eardrum 14 years ago.

Examination

On examination he has swollen inguinal lymph nodes bilaterally. Over the tip, in the sulcus and along the shaft of the penis he has groups of small ulcers. His temperature is 37.1°C.

INVESTIGATIONS
Swabs from the base of the genital lesion are desirable for proper diagnosis, counselling and management. However, in the area in which this GP worked, the facilities were not available for investigation and so diagnosis had to be made on clinical signs only.

Questions

- What is the diagnosis?
- He is very worried and cannot understand why his ex-wife denies having any symptoms. Can you explain this to him?
- What complications might arise?
- What do you advise him?

ANSWER

The patient has genital herpes. *Herpes simplex virus* type 1 is the usual cause of cold sores around the mouth and causes up to half the cases of genital herpes. *Herpes simplex virus* type 2 causes genital herpes and sometimes cold sores. At least half of those who develop genital herpes caught the virus from a sexual partner who was asymptomatic so the patient's ex-wife is likely to be telling the truth. There may be a connection between his history of cold sores and this present outbreak.

Complications include: local spread; extragenital spread to the buttocks, fingers or eye (in about 20 per cent of cases); aseptic meningitis in up to 20 per cent of patients with a first herpes simplex infection, with around 5 per cent of these patients needing hospitalization; hyperaesthesia; difficulties in micturition or defaecation; erythema multiforme; monoarthritis; hepatitis; thrombocytopenia; and superinfection with bacteria or *Candida*.

Because the herpes lesions developed more than 5 days previously and there are now no new lesions developing, oral antiviral medication (which stops the virus from replicating rather than clearing the virus from the body) will not be successful in limiting severity and duration of symptoms. The GP needs to explain this to the patient. The GP can recommend regular pain-killers, salt baths if the patient has a bath (half a cup of salt in the bath water), ice packs and plenty of fluids. The patient can be told that there may be recurrences but that they are usually less severe and of a shorter duration and that, if the lesions do return, to see a doctor or the local sexual health clinic for swabs and antiviral treatment as early as possible.

 KEY POINTS

- It is important to know or find out about the natural history and treatment of common infectious diseases.
- Giving wrong information, for example about a sexually transmitted infection, could cause unnecessary distress for a couple.
- Where possible, proper diagnosis should be made, with referral to the local sexual health clinic if necessary.
- Look on the internet if you need more information. Good websites are those of the British Association of Dermatologists, American Academy of Dermatology, New Zealand Dermatological Society, and DermAtlas.

CASE 85: SORE SHOULDER

History

The GP is visited by a 65-year-old woman with a 2-month history of a sore and stiff right shoulder. There is no history of injury. She is finding sleeping and dressing particularly difficult. It is also hard for her to brush her hair, pick up her grandchildren, carry the laundry basket, cook, make the bed, do the housework or travel on the bus: all her activities of daily living have been affected. A few months previously she had been mugged outside her door and had her handbag stolen and she feels very nervous about going outdoors, even more so since her shoulder injury. She lives alone in a one-bedroom flat which is on the ground floor of a big city estate. Her husband died a year previously. Her daughter and three young grandchildren live close by. She is still very tearful about losing her husband and has been sleeping poorly and not looking after her health. She has been tending to sit in her living room for most of the day. Her daughter has been helping her and it was she who persuaded her mother to go to her GP. The patient has not been to her general practice for some months since her yearly flu vaccine with the practice nurse. She has also seen a locum GP in the past year with a chest infection. Her GP has not seen her since her husband died. In the course of the conversation about her shoulder it becomes obvious that she is grieving and not coping well at home quite separately from the problems with her shoulder.

Examination

Her GP examines the shoulder and finds that there is limitation to abduction of the shoulder and external rotation at the shoulder on the right and considerable pain on these movements. These restrictions to movement occur whether the arm is being moved actively (by the patient) or passively (by the GP). Otherwise, there are no other obvious physical symptoms and the rest of her musculoskeletal examination is normal apart from a slightly stiff and painful neck. The rest of her physical examination is normal.

INVESTIGATIONS
The GP orders an X-ray of the affected shoulder and some blood tests, including blood glucose.

Questions

- What could be wrong with her shoulder and how do we make the diagnosis?
- What treatments are available for her shoulder injury?
- How can she be helped with her bereavement?

ANSWER

> The differential diagnosis includes adhesive capsulitis and degenerative glenohumeral arthritis.

The diagnosis in this case is thought to be adhesive capsulitis, which occurs in 2–4 per cent of adults and usually in middle age, rarely under 40 years or in the elderly and equally in males and females. In 20 per cent of people it is bilateral either concurrently or sequentially. The condition goes through three phases: the initial freezing stage which is very painful, the frozen stage where movement is limited and pain is less, and then the thawing stage where recovery occurs. Each stage can last months to a year and the final range of movement is often reduced. The pain is often referred to the upper outer arm around the deltoid. The cause is unknown, the process of disease being thickening and contraction of the shoulder joint capsule giving restricted range of movement. The intracapsular volume shrinks (5–10 mL volume rather than 20–30 mL). It affects external rotation particularly (then abduction and internal rotation) and both active and passive movements are affected (differs from other conditions). There are functional difficulties in daily tasks, such as grooming hair, buttoning up clothes, etc. Twenty per cent of people who suffer from this condition have diabetes.

Treatments can be provided at three levels: physical, psychological and social. On a physical level, medication can include simple analgesics such as paracetamol and non-steroidal anti-inflammatory drugs (NSAIDs) but be careful where there is a history of indigestion or peptic ulceration or asthma. Physiotherapy or steroid injections can sometimes be effective. Occasionally, manipulation under general anaesthetic is tried. The patient does need psychological support through family and friends, her GP and practice staff. A home help can give assistance with getting in and out of bed, washing, getting dressed and undressed, going to the toilet, eating meals, shopping, collecting benefits/pension, preparing meals, essential household tasks and laundry. Occupational therapy, for example, can help by providing equipment and adaptations to the home but in the UK this is generally only provided by social services for long-term disability.

Bereavement counselling can be provided by her GP, practice counsellor, local mental health services (for the over 65s there can be a special mental health of older adults service) or bereavement counsellors (for example, in the UK, Cruse Bereavement Care can provide counselling and support from trained volunteers and is a free service).

 KEY POINTS

- It is very important to take a good history and make a thorough examination to properly evaluate her shoulder injury. Knowledge of the anatomy of the shoulder needs to be related to function, diagnosis and treatment.
- A reminder that when you consider a scenario such as this patient's think about her not as a medical case but a person with a sore shoulder and physical, psychological and social needs.
- Decisions on the diagnosis and treatment need to be made in the context of her psychological and social well-being.
- A seemingly minor problem for some is actually a major problem for an elderly woman living on her own in an inner city area.

History

A 34-year-old woman attends her GP with a sore throat associated with other symptoms of an upper respiratory tract infection. She also reports a long history of headaches, muscle aches and pains, palpitations and sleeplessness. She has attended the surgery a few times before for minor illnesses. From talking with her and from the medical notes the GP finds out that she is an asylum seeker from Somalia, recently granted refugee status in the UK, who came to the UK 6 years previously. Her first language is Kibajuni, she speaks some Somali and her English is basic: she is able to make herself understood by the GP but a more in-depth conversation about her health is not possible. However, from reading the notes it appears that she fled from Somalia after her husband and mother were killed and that she was raped during factional fighting. She made her way to the UK, via Kenya, and with the support of the Somali community has set up home in London. She lives with a Somali family and helps in the home and with the children. From taking a simple history and examining the patient, the sore throat appears to be viral in origin and the GP advises the woman to take paracetamol, drink plenty of fluids and avoid exertion for a few days. However, the woman is tearful and unhappy and the GP is concerned about her. She is not very forthcoming but is willing to return to talk more about her health, in particular about her physical symptoms and sleeplessness.

Questions

- What are possible causes of her headaches and sleeplessness?
- How might the GP find out more about what is going on?
- What would be helpful to explore in the initial assessments?
- What services would be of assistance in further assessment and treatment?

ANSWER

> There may be a physical cause of her headaches and sleeplessness but the most likely cause is a mental health problem.

The GP and the patient require an interpreter. The patient does not have family in London. She does have friends in her community who speak good English but the GP suspects that she wants to talk about private matters that she would not wish her friends to know about. The GP also would rather have a trained interpreter who is not known to the patient: the patient is happy with this. There are two types of interpreting services that the GP could also use. Telephone interpreting is available in the GP's area but on investigating, there is no Kibujani interpreter available. The woman is not keen to talk with an interpreter that is not from her tribal group because of what she experienced at the hands of another group. However there is a trained Kibujani interpreter at the local interpreting service who could attend with the patient at another appointment. They agree to meet again to talk in 2 weeks time and the GP asks her reception staff to book the interpreter for a 30-minute appointment at the end of a surgery to give time for the consultation.

The GP has heard about the results of a recent study that revealed that the most common mental health problems suffered by Somali refugees are depression and anxiety with 14 per cent suffering post-traumatic stress disorder (PTSD). The GP also finds out from the internet that such patients might not access health care or reveal mental health problems for fear of being stigmatized by their community, a common perception being that mental illness is incurable. The GP also learns that in Somalia there is a belief that it is best to not think about traumatic experiences and the patient may not like the idea of talking therapies. The Royal College of Psychiatrists has produced a leaflet on PTSD and the GP reads this.

The GP at the second consultation focuses on her mental health. After some discussion the GP, with the woman's agreement, refers her to the local community mental health team for initial assessment. Finally the GP arranges to meet with her and the interpreter in a month's time and they make another double appointment while the interpreter is present. At this appointment she plans to focus on the woman's physical health.

KEY POINTS

- Do one's homework and seek advice.
- Be aware of and sensitive to cultural beliefs.
- Think carefully about the most appropriate interpreter.
- The complexity of some patient's presentations may necessitate a number of consultations.
- Building trust is a prerequisite of effective care, especially in a patient who has suffered abuse in a situation where doctors and the state might not always be trustworthy.

CASE 87: SQUINT

History

The GP has been seeing a new mother with postnatal depression (see Case 56). She has just started counselling and is now on antidepressants and is starting to feel brighter. She comes along to the GP with her baby for the 6-week check and reports that she thinks that the baby may have a squint. Her husband had a squint in childhood that required two operations. As a result of his squint being treated late he has no binocular vision and has severely reduced vision in his affected eye. He is particularly concerned about the baby.

For the first few weeks the baby's eyes did wander and, as this can be normal in a new baby, they were advised not to be worried about it. However, the parents have noticed that the baby's right eye does now appear to be able to focus on things but the baby's left eye left tends to slide inwards.

The baby was born distressed at 36 weeks after a long labour and was in the Special Care Baby Unit for a few days and discharged in good health. Since then the baby has been well and is being bottle-fed as the mother could not cope with breast-feeding because she had been feeling so low and out of touch with her baby. The health visitor has been seeing the family regularly and has noticed an improvement in the bonding with the baby over the past week or so.

Questions

- What are some of the causes of a squint?
- How would the GP examine the baby?
- What should the GP do next?

ANSWER

A squint may be intermittent because of the baby's immature visual system, resolving by about 4 months or congenital (usually esotropic or a convergent squint); in an older child (usually 2 years or older) it may be caused by refractive errors. It may occasionally be caused by infection, prematurity, neurological disorder (for example hydrocephalus or cerebral palsy) or brain injury; very rarely, it is caused by a tumour such as a retinoblastoma.

It is not easy to examine a baby's eyes. What looks like a squint can be caused by the shape of the eyes and wide medial epicanthal folds. The corneal light reflex can be seen at arms' length without unduly disturbing the child: with a true squint the corneal light reflex is asymmetrical. The cover test is a little more difficult and may not be possible in such a young baby: the GP covers the eye that looks normal and then watches the uncovered abnormal-looking eye for movement as it takes up fixation. An important part of the examination is the red reflex using the ophthalmoscope set at '0' at a distance of about 25 cm. A cataract or corneal opacity will show up as black against the red reflex and fundal lesions will appear white. In addition, as always, the GP must take into account the baby's general health.

In this situation the baby has a number of risk factors for a squint: she was born prematurely (before 37 weeks) and has a family history of squint. The GP does find an obvious convergent squint in the left eye. Even though the baby is younger than the normal age a referral would be made for a possible squint, the GP, because of the risk factors, makes the decision to refer the baby to the local orthoptic clinic. The baby is seen and a congenital squint is diagnosed. The orthoptist refers the baby to an ophthalmologist and surgery is carried out to correct this squint. In other situations spectacles can be used to correct sight problems in older children, and occlusion can also be used, patching the good eye to encourage the weaker eye to be used.

 KEY POINTS

- As a rule, the younger a child's squint can be corrected the quicker and greater the improvement in vision.
- Where there is a family history of squint or a constant squint at the 6- to 8-week baby check, referral should be made.
- If the squint is not treated until the child is over 6–11 years old normal vision cannot usually be restored.

History

Your next patient has led a troubled life. She is a 47-year-old divorced woman, who has worked variously as a hairdresser, a shop assistant and a building society clerk. She now lives alone since her three children have grown up and left; the children have different fathers, which in her case reflects her difficulty in making or keeping relationships. She uses a salbutamol inhaler intermittently for asthma, not helped by her smoking five to ten cigarettes a day. She is overweight (body mass index 28), and has a tendency to reflux oesophagitis more or less contained by alginate-antacid (Gaviscon) and a proton-pump inhibitor (lansoprazole). She also complains from time to time of musculoskeletal pains, for which she has in the past been prescribed co-proxamol. She drinks, by her account, 20 units a week, but you have long suspected it is considerably more.

She has been attending more frequently in the last year, with lethargy, headache and insomnia. She denies feeling depressed, but her somatic symptoms, the expression on her face, her downcast gaze and apathetic voice all speak otherwise. What she really wants is a sleeping-pill, such as the Mogadon she used to use.

Questions

- What further questions might you ask her?
- What treatment might help her?
- How would you monitor her progress?

ANSWER

You ask her directly 'Have you ever felt as if life is not worth living?' When she says yes, you ask 'Have you ever tried to harm yourself?' She denies suicidal feelings, and you think she might be amenable to a combination of antidepressant therapy and some behavioural therapy. You offer her an appointment with the practice counsellor, and offer a prescription for citalopram. But she says she had these a few months ago and stopped taking them because they worsened her indigestion, and did nothing for her insomnia. Instead, you give her a small quantity (20 tablets) of amitriptyline, 25 mg daily. You ask her to see you again in 2 weeks; you make a note that she may need referral to the local mental health team.

The following Monday, you take a phone call from the Coroner's Office: your patient was admitted to hospital over the weekend having taken a mixed overdose of co-proxamol (apparently saved from old prescriptions), amitriptyline and alcohol. She died from a cardiac arrest, despite intensive therapy. At the subsequent inquest, the Coroner finds that she took her own life, and you are relieved to find no public blame attaches to you.

 KEY POINTS

- Most suicidal patients will have contacted their doctor with a week or two of their attempt, but most patients who visit their doctors are not suicidal. Spotting the high-risk patient (the 'signal in the noise') is a large part of the art of medicine. Contrary to common belief, careful enquiry into the patient's thoughts about suicide does not increase the risk.
- Dextropropoxyphene, an opioid drug, rapidly causes potentially fatal abnormal heart rhythms and respiratory depression when taken in overdose and has now been withdrawn from the market in the UK. The combination of alcohol with paracetamol, exacerbated by dextropropoxyphene (as in co-proxamol), is well known to be potentially lethal.
- Despite recent critical comment, serotonin-reuptake inhibitors remain much safer in overdose than tricyclics which can trigger cardiac arrhythmias unpredictably.
- Even (especially) your 'failures' can teach you much. In this case, perhaps a greater readiness to involve a mental health team at an earlier stage could have offered this vulnerable patient support at what, with hindsight, was a critical stage in her life.

CASE 89: SWOLLEN ANKLES

History

Your next patient has survived pretty well, reaching the age of 88 years and still independent. As she says, bits of her body don't always obey orders, but thanks to your treatment she manages. Her osteoarthritis is mostly controlled with paracetamol, occasionally boosted by diclofenac. Her atrial fibrillation has made her breathless in the past, but has been well controlled with a pulse around 80 beats/minute, by taking a modest dose of digoxin. She rarely needs to use the glyceryl trinitrate inhaler, especially since her neighbour has been helping with the garden. Her incipient heart failure had been eased by taking a low-dose thiazide diuretic each morning. She maintains the standards of speech, courtesy, dress and comportment of a different age, and is still able to complete the *Daily Telegraph* crossword puzzle every day, though it takes her longer now. You would never dream of addressing her by her first name. But she is now troubled by swollen ankles; this is despite her electric recliner chair, bought by her daughter.

Examination

She has definite bilateral oedema, extending up to mid-shins. Her pulse rate remains the same, still slightly irregular; her blood pressure is 160/95 mmHg, which may not fulfil the strictest criteria but probably serves to pump the blood well enough through her gradually sclerosing circulation. You decide to increase her bendroflumethiazide, from 2.5 to 5 mg daily, and ask her to return in a month. When she does, you are disappointed to find no significant improvement; and her breathlessness is increasing.

Questions

- Why is she not improving?
- What can, or should, you do about it?

ANSWER

You try again, this time using furosemide 20 mg daily. But a week later you have to visit her at home, because of worsening breathlessness. This time she has an obvious chest infection and you prescribe some antibiotics. You give her a starter dose from your bag and have to go to the kitchen for a glass of water to help her swallow it. There, you find in a cupboard, boxes of unused tablets – the diuretics you have been prescribing assiduously for months. She has not taken more than half a dozen of them. When you ask her, she is embarrassed to admit that she found them too efficacious; she would have to rush to the toilet, and her arthritis slowed her down, so that she had the occasional 'accident'. She did not want to offend you, so she continued to accept your prescription, and merely put the pills to one side.

You suggest that she try to take a half-dose, say twice a day (morning and mid-day), as you think it would help her breathlessness, even if she is not troubled by the ankle swelling. She agrees to this, at least on a short-term basis.

 KEY POINTS

- Think of the consequences of taking medication: not just side-effects, but the very effects themselves may be worse for a patient than the disease.
- For many older patients, the prospect of dying holds little terror; loss of dignity is far more serious. As doctors, we may have to compromise on scientific exactitude and accept our patient's needs on their terms.

CASE 90: TIREDNESS

History

Billy is an active 11-year-old, who lives in a busy normal family. His mother brings him in with vague symptoms: he is not eating as well as usual, he is getting tired and his school-work is deteriorating. His medical records show the normal minor ailments of childhood, but no serious illnesses. You know his mother well: she has chronic anxiety and depression, and takes citalopram, with some benefit.

Examination

He seems lively enough, alert, though perhaps a little pale next to his robust mother. He is wary of the stethoscope and fearful you might give him an injection. You can find nothing else of note on examination, and suspect that his illness is a cover for an exacerbation of his mother's hypochondriacal symptoms.

 INVESTIGATIONS

You advise a blood test, but he objects, as he does not like needles. His mother asks if it is really necessary. You persuade them to go ahead, and arrange to see him next week. The laboratory phones you next day with the results: haemoglobin 9.5 g/dL, leucocyte count 24×10^9/L, with morphology indicating acute lymphocytic leukaemia.

Questions

- What is your next step?
- What can they expect to happen?
- What can you tell his mother about prognosis?

ANSWER

You do not wait for the booked appointment. You phone his mother, tell her the blood test shows 'anaemia', and ask her to bring him to see you that evening. You then tell them the diagnosis, explain that he will need to see a paediatrician, who will probably arrange for admission and treatment. You phone the duty paediatric registrar, who advises that they come to the outpatients department next day. You type out the referral letter and give it to mother by hand.

Billy may need to be admitted for a blood transfusion, and will have to have a cocktail of medicines to induce remission (stop his marrow producing the leukaemia cells). Some of his treatment will be as an inpatient, but mostly he will be attending the outpatient clinic. He may need maintenance therapy for several years. He may have side-effects, such as sickness or hair loss. The problem of gonadal damage is complex, and you decide to leave that to the paediatric oncology team.

Survival rates for acute leukaemia are improving all the time, and Billy stands a better than 80 per cent chance of beating his disease. His care is absorbed by the hospital 'machine', but a month later you see him, pinker and fitter, tolerating his drug regime equably, and with a fashionable short haircut. That Christmas, you receive a card from Billy, with a grateful note from his mother.

 KEY POINTS

- With hindsight, why did you insist on the blood test, against the patient's first wishes? The decision can be rationalized ('he had pallor; his tiredness was unusual for him'), but often spotting the 'signal' of serious disease in the background 'noise' of routine minor ailments is instinctive, based on experience and a hunch.
- Build up your database of minor illnesses based on your daily routine, so that when you do see a sick person, you can identify them, even if you cannot at first identify their illness.

History

'I feel tired all the time'. Your next patient looks and sounds as tired as she feels. She is a 63-year-old school dinner lady, married, with one daughter married, who has been treated in the past for arthritic joint pains and still takes occasional diclofenac and paracetamol. She has a dull complexion, mousy hair, lacklustre clothes, a downcast expression and a subdued voice. She says she has felt tired for nearly a year, and has put it down to the demands of her job and housework. Her periods stopped about 8 years ago. Her appetite is normal, though she does not really enjoy food now. She is a non-smoker and rarely drinks. She has no problems passing urine, but admits to constipation, and has to take Senna from time to time. Her weight is stable. Her sleep has been disordered recently with early-morning waking. Questions about her family reveal no sensitive topics, though she is busy at home caring for her own mother who has mild dementia and a colostomy.

Examination

Examination, including a rectal examination, reveals nothing of note. Her weight is as usual with a body mass index of 27. Her pulse rate, blood pressure, heart and lungs, and abdomen all appear normal.

INVESTIGATIONS
A full blood count, renal function and thyroid function tests are normal.

Questions

- Is there a diagnosis to fit this clinical picture?
- How would you like to treat this patient?

ANSWER

> Anaemia, caused by her long-term consumption of a non-steroidal anti-inflammatory drug, is ruled out by the normal blood count. Hypothyroidism is not supported by her normal thyroid function test. Renal failure is also ruled out by normal renal function tests. There are no menopausal symptoms: no hot flushes or night sweats or vaginal dryness. She certainly has features suggestive of depression.

You decide to give her citalopram, 20 mg daily, and she shows considerable improvement, looking and feeling brighter within a month.

However, the constipation persists, despite taking regular ispaghula fibre and lactulose. Her erythrocyte sedimentation rate (ESR) is slightly raised, at 35 mm/hour. An abdominal scan shows no obvious abnormality. The constipation persists and you pay more attention to her family history. You decide to refer her for colonoscopy, which reveals a descending colon neoplasm. Fortunately, it is still restricted to the lumen, and she is able to have an end-to-end anastomosis, thus avoiding a stoma herself.

 KEY POINTS

- Patients can have more than one diagnosis: Ockham's Razor ('keep it simple') does not always apply in medical diagnosis.
- If a symptom does not fit your original diagnosis, or does not respond to your treatment, consider an alternative: have a 'Plan B', in case 'Plan A' fails.
- And an occult faecal blood test might have helped in this case.

CASE 92: TIREDNESS

History

The GP is consulted by a 25-year-old woman who consults infrequently. She is a strong believer in alternative medicine and attends a homeopath and nutritionist for her usual health care. Her nutritionist has asked her to see the GP as they think that she is in the early stages of hypothyroidism. Privately done blood tests have revealed thyroxine (T4) and triiodothyronine (T3) on the lower side of normal with a normal thyroid stimulating hormone (TSH) level and a normal full blood count. The patient tells the GP that she has been feeling tired recently. She works as a yoga teacher and lives with her boyfriend in a rented flat that they have shared for 2 years. She is a vegetarian and eats well. Her health has previously been good and she is on no medication. She uses condoms for contraception and is not keen to use any allopathic medication. She does attend for regular smears. She says that she has been feeling tired off and on over the past 4 months and a little bit down. It is now March and she thinks that she does suffer from mild seasonal affective disorder. She has also been working very hard as her and her boyfriend want to buy a house and she has not had a holiday since the previous July. Her boyfriend has been away a lot as he travels as part of his work with a charity. She does not have any other symptoms although she has had two upper respiratory tract infections over the winter, which is unusual for her. Specifically, apart from the tiredness and mild depression she does not have symptoms of dry hair and skin, constipation, weight gain or feeling unusually cold, other symptoms suggestive of an underactive thyroid. She has not had any previous serious illness. Her maternal aunt does have hypothyroidism and her maternal grandmother has maturity-onset Type 2 diabetes. There is no other family history of note. She tells you that her and her boyfriend would like to try for a baby once they have bought a house. Her periods are regular. She has not been pregnant or tried for a pregnancy. She does not smoke.

Examination

Examination is normal.

Questions

- How does the GP approach this situation?
- What more does the GP need to know?
- What should the GP do further?

ANSWER

A respectful approach is required. Even if the GP thinks differently to the patient and her therapist about alternative medicine there is no point alienating her or undermining her relationship with her therapist unless the GP thinks that the patient is being seriously damaged by her actions. After discussion with her and explaining that he does not think that she has hypothyroidism the GP agrees to her request to repeat her thyroid function through the local NHS hospital laboratory. He also repeats her full blood count and checks her ferritin, folic acid and vitamin B_{12} levels, although he is pretty sure that her diet is good and that these will be normal. The results do come back as normal with low normal T3 and T4 levels, and a normal TSH level. Thyroid antibody levels are normal. The patient gives the GP permission to ring and speak with the nutritionist to whom he explains his findings. The nutritionist does think that the young woman is at risk of hypothyroidism and tells the GP that she will keep an eye on the situation and refer the woman back to him if there are any developments. There is also a suggestion of mild clinical depression but the patient is not willing to explore this further with the GP and says that she will look for solutions to this elsewhere.

 KEY POINTS

- It is important to work with and respect your patient even if you might have different opinions.
- One of your roles as an allopathic doctor is to present your findings and understandings, if requested, to patients and alternative practitioners.
- Bear in mind that, in the long term, the alternative practitioner might be right and the patient may develop hypothyroidism.

History

Your next consultation involves a reluctant patient, brought by his mother because she thinks he is more tired than usual. He is 17 years old, attends a local college where he is learning business studies, and he does not think he has a medical problem. His mother has noticed that in the last 6 months or so he has had difficulty getting up in the morning to go to college, has fallen asleep while doing his homework, and is not taking part in football or any sports as much as before. She also thinks his appetite is worse.

Examination

He has a pallid complexion, a body mass index of 19, and a scattering of acne across his back. He cooperates reasonably with the consultation and examination, but you can find no remarkable signs except some vaguely defined lymph nodes palpable in his neck.

Questions

- Do his symptoms represent a departure from the normal pattern?
- What further information would you like to obtain from him?
- How would you manage this case?

ANSWER

The lethargic youth is a stereotype, and this patient may merely be 'passing through a phase', but you need more information before coming to this conclusion. Consider the possibility of alcohol and drug abuse. You have already noted the absence of suspicious marks around his veins, and the normal reactions of his pupils. You need to see him on his own, either by asking mother to leave, or by arranging another appointment. You can then ask about his use of recreational drugs: cannabis is quite likely, but he may be reluctant to admit to using other agents such as ecstasy or cocaine. Careful enquiry as to his sexual habits would be useful in case he is at risk of *Human immunodeficiency virus* (HIV) infection. In the course of your consultation, you can assess whether he seems to have unusual patterns of thought or speech, suggesting the possibility of an early schizophrenic disorder.

All these findings are negative. Although reserved in manner, he does not appear particularly depressed. He has been losing a little weight lately, which is unusual in a growing youth. A repeat examination of his lymph glands confirms your earlier impression, although he has no signs of an enlarged liver or spleen. A blood test shows a haemoglobin of 10.3 g/dL, and a lymphocytosis; a glandular fever screen is negative. In view of his weight loss, anaemia and swollen glands, you refer him urgently to the haematologist. After scans (including a positron-emission tomography, or PET, scan) and lymph gland biopsy, the diagnosis of Hodgkin's lymphoma is confirmed, and the young man starts on a course of chemotherapy, with good prospects of a complete cure.

 KEY POINTS

- Stereotypes are deceptive friends. Every formal diagnosis is a stereotype, but each patient is individual.
- Careful physical examination is necessary with all patients with a physical complaint.
- When we suspect psychological problems, we should look for positive features of psychological disorder before making a psychological diagnosis. Conversely, the mere absence of major physical signs does not mean the absence of physical disease.

History

A 73-year-old man presents to his GP because he has problems sleeping. Further enquiry reveals that he has to get up four to five times at night to pass urine in the last year: 'I have always been a light sleeper and getting back to sleep can be a real struggle'. The GP continues to take a history of the patient's urinary symptoms. The patient admits that starting urination has been delayed more often and the stream of urine is not as strong at the end, causing some dribbling. At night times especially he feels he has not been able to empty the bladder completely. The patient says that it has become more difficult to hold urine and when he starts feeling the need to urinate he has to go and find a toilet immediately. He has limited his car journeys and has identified toilets in town not to get caught out. The doctor proceeds to do a rectal examination and finds an evenly enlarged prostate with a diminished central sulcus. The gland feels smooth and is not tender. 'You seem to have developed an enlarged prostate. This is common when you get older and it's not cancer. I will need to arrange further blood tests to confirm my finding. I can start you on medication to improve your symptoms. Here is a leaflet explaining it all', says the doctor handing over the paper together with the prescription of the prostate drug.

The patient seems to be slow getting up from his chair: 'Is there anything you have not understood?' asks the doctor. At the door the patient the patient says 'No you have been really good to explain it doctor. Thank you. It's just that the sore on my tongue has not disappeared yet'. The GP tells the patient to take a seat again and checks the records. His colleague entered a clinical note 4 weeks ago that reads 'suspicious looking ulcer on lateral border of the tongue. Smoked pipe for 40 years. Review in 2 weeks and consider urgent referral if no better'.

Questions
• Why did the patient delay presenting his main concern until the end of the consultation?
• Who is responsible for the delay in following up a suspicious lesion?

ANSWER

Given the last entry in the records the patient might quite reasonably have expected the GP to ask questions about the tongue ulcer. From the notes it is not clear how much the patient has been told and if he has been made aware of the potentially malignant nature of his condition. There is a danger that patients and doctors collude when new, potentially serious symptoms arise. The doctor would prefer not to give bad news and the patient has really come for reassurance. This danger increases when doctor and patient are old friends, sharing a close relationship.

Patients, especially the elderly, do not want to be a nuisance to doctors. Sometimes they are not sure if their suffering is severe enough to warrant medical attention. At other times the symptoms are so personal and potentially embarrassing that it is difficult to present them. A common coping mechanism in this situation it to test the waters first, seeing if the doctor is sympathetic towards them and building up confidence through the consultation. Symptoms presented can be minor such as a rash or a cough, seen by the public as 'medical'. The public copes with an enormous amount of untreated symptoms and disease. This gentleman's urinary symptoms had been bothering him for at least a year.

Patients often gives clues about the topic they are really interested in and, if all else fails, disclose their real concern when they are about to leave the room. It can be tempting for doctors to dismiss a concern brought forward by patients leaving the room. In this case, the doctor is likely to have spent more than the 10 minutes allocated and might feel under pressure trying to catch up on time. A reasonable compromise can be to clarify the concern and ask the patient to return if the matter is not urgent.

The doctor who saw the patient presenting with the suspicious tongue ulcer identified the appropriate length of time for review for the patient and documented his concerns well. However, he failed to specify and document who was responsible arranging the review. Most likely he would have asked the patient to make an appointment in 2 weeks time if the ulcer had not disappeared. In practices that do not allow booking of appointments in advance it can be difficult, especially for elderly patients, to gain access.

 KEY POINTS

- Patients sometimes test the water first before presenting their most important complaint.
- A skilled listener can be alerted to this by watching out for clues given by the patient. Never dismiss a complaint raised by a patient leaving the room before you have clarified what is wrong.
- It is the doctor's responsibility to be clear to patients and in the clinical notes about follow-up arrangements for potentially serious illnesses.

History

The GP is visited by a 68-year-old man and his wife, both long-time patients of the surgery. For the past few months the man has noticed that his left hand has been shaking. This is worse in the morning. He is left-handed, and a keen bowls player, and his symptoms are now getting in the way of his game. He and his wife live in a council house on the local estate where they have lived since they were married, 40 years ago. They brought up their three children there who are now married with children. The man worked for the post office and his wife was a care assistant. They have been retired for the past 3 years and have enjoyed their retirement, looking after their grandchildren, playing bowls and visiting their youngest son and his family who live in Scotland. The patient has been generally well although he has developed benign prostatic hypertrophy which is being followed by the urologists.

Questions

- What is the differential diagnosis where there is a tremor?
- What should the GP focus on in the history and examination?
- What does the GP do next?

ANSWER

A physiological tremor, where all other examination is normal, is a low-amplitude, fine tremor. The tremor is common in thyrotoxicosis and can be enhanced by drugs and toxins such as lithium carbonate, bronchodilators, caffeine, lead, arsenic and carbon monoxide.

Essential tremor, the most common form of tremor, is predominantly a postural or action-type tremor with about 50 per cent of sufferers having a positive family history. It is temporarily reduced by alcohol and can affect any part of the body.

Parkinson's tremor is a low-frequency tremor at rest, disappearing with action. If it occurs in the hand it may appear as the classic 'pill rolling' tremor of thumb and forefinger. This may also occur as a result of Wilson's disease, heavy metal poisoning or anti-psychotic medication.

An intention tremor is low-frequency, occurs during activity and is often more marked as the limb nears the target. It can be caused by a cerebellar lesion as a result, for example, of multiple sclerosis, cerebellar injury or stroke, or as a result of toxins such as alcohol.

The GP focuses on history and examination that differentiates between the causes of the tremor. The patient has also felt very tired, and a bit stiff and slow in his movements and his handwriting has been getting spidery. The GP suspects that this patient might have Parkinson's disease. To be diagnosed with Parkinson's he needs to have two of the three symptoms of tremor, rigidity and bradykinesia and he reports all three with a one-sided tremor at rest that disappears with action.

The patient is referred and the neurologist makes a diagnosis of Parkinson's disease and prescribes Sinemet (levodopa and carbidopa) that has a good effect on his functioning. Fortunately, the local hospital has a multidisciplinary consultation clinic delivering a model of care fitting the National Institute for Health and Clinical Excellence (NICE) guidelines. The team provides rapid access to consultant-led specialist care and assessment and includes physiotherapists, occupational therapists, speech and language specialists as well as access to psychological and psychiatric support. The patient receives regular review, 3- to 6-monthly, and medication advice and becomes part of an expert patient group. He has a specialist nurse who leads his care and is available to him and his wife and the GP when they need advice.

 KEY POINTS

- Parkinson's disease is a condition diagnosed primarily on history and examination.
- Rapid referral to an expert is required for accurate diagnosis and specialized care.
- Patient-centred care and multidisciplinary support is essential for this condition.

CASE 96: UNEXPLAINED SYMPTOMS

History

Your next patient is a 27-year-old Central African man, who speaks better French than English, and better Kikongo than both. He works as a driver, and has come to see you with a slightly embarrassing problem. Recently, he has noticed that after making love, he experiences a curious metallic taste in his mouth, and a general bodily weakness. He has a long-standing relationship with a woman from his home country, and he says he has not been unfaithful, and does not think she has either. They have no children as yet. Apart from this singular symptom, he says his general health is good; he enjoys swimming and football, and certainly appears in good physical health. He says he has had no discharge from the penis, and his partner has no vaginal problems. He is on no medication.

Examination

His blood pressure is 110/70 mmHg, his heart and lungs sound normal. A careful inspection of his mouth and dentition reveals nothing unusual. He has no surgical scars or other abdominal abnormalities. His testicles are normal, his penis (circumcised when he was a child) likewise, with no evidence of rash, sores or discharge.

 INVESTIGATIONS

You discuss with him the problems associated with testing for *Human immunodeficiency virus*, and he agrees to a blood test to include this, a treponemal test for syphilis, a blood count, sickle cell screen and a blood glucose check. You also take a urethral swab, including a *Chlamydia* test. When you see him next week, all of these tests are normal.

Questions

- Should you reassure or refer him?
- How much further investigation is indicated?

He tells you that since his last visit, his partner has consulted her doctor (not in the same practice), and has had her contraceptive hormone implant removed from her arm. Subsequently, after sexual relations, he now does not notice the symptom, and he thinks it is as a result of the removal of the implant. You tell him that you are pleased he is better, and you can assure him that your own examination and tests have shown no abnormality; indeed, he seems in the best of health. However, you have no explanation for his symptoms. Seeking a possible psychosomatic cause, you ask if there have been any other difficulties with his girlfriend. He is puzzled by this, and it is clear he and his partner have a generally untroubled relationship. He does not indicate any dissatisfaction with his sexual performance. Since he is better, you decide to leave him alone, and simply ask him to return if the problem recurs. You suggest he may wish to bring his partner if he does return to you. The case remains unsolved.

KEY POINTS

- Not every problem in general practice is amenable to a final diagnosis. You may have to limit yourself to a description of symptoms, signs and investigations in puzzling cases. Living with uncertainty is part of a GP's lot.
- Not every undiagnosed problem needs referral. The symptoms may be trivial, and if serious disease is not suspected, can be left alone unless the patient becomes increasingly worried.
- You may wish, in unsolved cases, to seek advice from colleagues, from the library or from the internet. If these are unsuccessful, you may even consider writing it up to send to a journal as a clinical curiosity.

CASE 97: UNUSUAL BEHAVIOUR

History

Your patient has had difficulties for years. He is now 22 years old, and has moderately severe schizophrenia. He functions at a basic level, living alone but supported by a network of social and mental health-care workers. His life has been punctuated by admissions to the psychiatric unit, but provided that he continues to receive his regular injections of fluphenazine from the community mental health nurse, and remembers to take his daily orphenadrine, he remains tolerably well and cheerful. When he claims to receive broadcasts in his head from the BBC, and behaves in bizarre ways, it is time to ask for an urgent review by the psychiatrist. He does not work, and his principal pleasure in life is eating, so much so that he is now very obese.

After a quiet interval of some months, your receptionist receives a phone call from his neighbour, asking for the doctor to call as the patient cannot walk to the surgery. When you call at his flat, you have difficulty gaining entrance. Peering through the letter-box, you see him on the floor, trying to walk on his hands and knees. Eventually, he gets to the front door and opens it, staggering back to sit again on the floor. This is even more bizarre behaviour than usual, and he is unable to give any history to account for it. He seems rather more confused than distressed, and you note the general disorder and decay of his home.

Questions

- What referral method would be appropriate here?
- What non-psychiatric causes can you suggest for these symptoms?

ANSWER

An urgent referral for psychiatric assessment would seem the first choice. If, as seems likely, he is unable to give informed consent to admission, you may need to invoke the Mental Health Act 1983. The usual course is to use Section 2, which requires a relative or social worker to sign an application form (Forms 1 or 2), and two doctors (GP and psychiatrist) to sign Form 3. This permits detention in a hospital unit for assessment for up to 28 days. If longer admission, or treatment, is needed, Section 3 is invoked. If time does not permit waiting for a psychiatrist, Section 4, requiring only a relative (Form 5) and the GP (Form 7) can be used for admission for up to 72 hours. The ambulance crew may request police support if the patient is likely to be opposed to admission. All of these can be harrowing experiences for the patient, and a voluntary admission is much preferred.

You may suspect a sudden onset of muscle weakness, possibly an extrapyramidal side-effect of his fluphenazine, or alternatively, in view of his obesity, a diabetic crisis previously unnoticed because of his irregular attendance at surgery.

In this case, you return to the surgery to arrange a Section 2 admission, but when the social worker arrives at the house, the patient is found to be dead on the floor. The inevitable Coroner's post-mortem examination reveals bilateral deep vein thromboses and a fatal pulmonary embolus. The verdict is death through natural causes, and no further action is taken.

 KEY POINTS

- Do not jump to conclusions: psychiatric patients can suffer physical illness, and the statistics show that they are more likely to experience physical ill health than the mentally stable population, and are more likely to have their illnesses misdiagnosed.
- Remember to examine patients appropriately: observation of severe breathlessness and examination of this patient's swollen legs could have led to life-saving treatment.
- Medical failures can be chastening, but we must learn from our mistakes not to repeat them.

History

The GP is visited by a new patient, a young woman of 21 years of age, and her mother. They are both looking glum and the young woman is slightly tearful. The young woman explains that she has recently had a miscarriage at 8 weeks gestation. The pregnancy was not planned but she and her boyfriend were very excited when they knew that she was pregnant and are now very upset about the loss. Her mother, who has three other grown-up children, is more philosophical although she is sad for her daughter and was looking forward to her second grandchild. The GP was not aware of the pregnancy and when she looks at the computer notes, sees that the patient had seen the locum 3 weeks before when she had missed her period and the pregnancy test was positive. The locum had referred her to the local antenatal clinic for early scanning and a booking appointment, with a request for shared care between the clinic and the practice. A few days before the present appointment the patient had started with some light bleeding that soon proceeded to uterine cramps and heavier bleeding with large clots. The heavy bleeding had lasted for about 6 hours through the night. In the morning her mother had taken her to the hospital Accident and Emergency Department where they had sent her to the early pregnancy assessment unit and a miscarriage was diagnosed. The bleeding is now very light and there are no pains or fever which might suggest that the miscarriage is incomplete. The girl's main concern is why the miscarriage happened and could there be something wrong with her or her boyfriend. Will she ever be able to have a baby? She likes to run; has this caused the miscarriage? They made love the night before the bleeding started; did this do some damage?

The patient tells the GP that she has been perfectly well; neither she or her partner have conceived before; she has been fully immunized. She does not smoke, her partner smokes occasionally and they are moderate drinkers, she drinking about 10 units of alcohol a week and he about 21, usually at the weekend. As far as she knows she does not have any hormonal or uterine problems or problems with her blood. Because the miscarriage was before 12 weeks, even if the patient is Rhesus negative she will not need Anti-D.

Examination

She appears of normal weight with a body mass index of 23 and her blood pressure is 110/68 mmHg. Abdominal examination is normal.

Questions
- What advice could the GP offer?

ANSWER

The GP explains that one in four pregnancies end in miscarriage and that usually it is very difficult to determine why the miscarriage happened, especially when it does so in the first trimester, as in this case. About half of early miscarriages occur because of an isolated chromosomal fault that rarely occurs again; miscarriage can also be caused by immunological, hormonal or anatomical problems, blood disorders or infection. It is very unlikely that the patient has a problem and investigations are not needed unless she has three or more miscarriages. The GP can reassure the patient that research has shown that doing moderate exercise or having sex while pregnant does not increase the risk of miscarriage.

The patient talks about wanting to have a child but needing time to get over the miscarriage. They had been using condoms and she decides to also use the progesterone-only pill for a few months. The GP suggests that she take folic acid daily to reduce the risk of fetal abnormalities were she to get pregnant. The GP also advises that she eats well, avoiding food such as soft cheeses, pâté, ready-prepared food, unless it is very well cooked, unpasteurized milk and raw or partially cooked eggs, drink little or no alcohol and limit caffeine intake. Because the patient had heavy bleeding with the miscarriage the GP suggests that she concentrate on eating iron-rich foods for the next few weeks, including green leafy vegetables, broccoli, dried fruit, wholegrain cereals, pulses and baked beans (she does not eat red meat), taken with food rich in vitamin C as this aids absorption. Finally exercising and getting plenty of sleep will help her recovery and general health. They make another appointment in 2 weeks.

 KEY POINTS

- The loss of a pregnancy can be devastating for a couple and sensitive counselling is vital.
- Patients can be reassured that miscarriage is common and is not caused by anything that they have done wrong or, in the majority of cases, anything that is wrong with them.

History

The practice nurse seeks advice from the GP about a 52-year-old diabetic woman who has come requesting sibutramine tablets to lose weight. She is well known to the practice nurse, but rarely sees the doctors in the practice. The nurse says 'I don't know what else I can do to help this patient' and she gives a summary of the patient. She has known her for 5 years when the patient was referred to the nurse for weight loss having been diagnosed with reduced fasting glucose tolerance. Her body mass index (BMI) was 31 and the nurse had provided advice on diet and exercise. The patient had returned for weighing after variable intervals. There had been a short period of success when the patient joined Weight Watchers, but over the years her weight had gone up rather than down and she reached a BMI of 35. Last year's fasting glucose test was even worse and she was diagnosed with diabetes. In order to help her to lose weight, she had been offered orlistat tablets, but failed to have any success, complaining of abdominal discomfort, distension, flatulence and diarrhoea. The patient had returned to the nurse 4 weeks ago requesting sibutramine, stating that her friend had managed to lose weight on this drug. The nurse had checked her blood pressure and pulse rate, stressing the patient must return after 2 weeks for another pulse and blood pressure check, but the patient had failed to attend. Now, 2 weeks late, with a weight loss of about 1 kg the patient has returned asking to have the dose of her tablets increased. 'I can't prescribe her the medication; it's against the guidelines not to have regular check-ups. She should have returned a fortnight ago. How can I continue prescribing? I really want to help her and she says she is motivated, but I don't seem to be getting anywhere. It gives me a dreadful sensation when I see this patient's name on my list. She makes me feel like a failure. Can you help?'

Questions
- How would you describe the nurse–patient relationship?
- What factors might be contributing to the patient's inability to lose weight?
- Are there any tests you would like to arrange?

ANSWER

The nurse–patient relationship has deteriorated. The nurse feels her heart 'sink' when she is asked to see the patient. At the same time the patient is likely to be unaware of the nurse's feelings. Years ago the nurse took charge, educating the patient about lifestyle hoping to help the patient. While happy to listen to the nurse's advice, the patient failed to lose weight. However, she continued to believe in the nurse and continued asking her to make her better, trying to make the nurse feel responsible for the situation. When the patient was diagnosed with diabetes she seemed to have become more motivated to commit to changes and the nurse started her on anti-obesity medication. However, the patient failed to take responsibility in turning up for her scheduled review appointment, making it difficult for the nurse to justify continuation of her medication.

Being overweight or obese stems from patients' inability to regulate food intake to the daily caloric requirements of the body. The lack of dietary control can be caused by different reasons. The nurse educated the patient about diet and exercise, energy contents of food and body requirements. This approach is highly successful if the main reason for being overweight is lack of knowledge. Often, patients do know about calories, diet, exercise and daily requirements, but feel unwilling or unable to make the necessary changes. Patient with busy lifestyles and long working hours claim not to have enough time to make the changes.

Some overweight patients lack insight and see themselves as having normal weight and this is more common when the rest of their family is obese. There are myths about obesity and some patients believe it is in their genes to be a good food converter and they have no choice but to become obese. Many overweight patients lack self-confidence and they can become victims of bullying. Patients who are emotionally upset can feel overwhelmed by the changes requested of their lives by health professionals, making them unable to engage in the treatment.

Patients with diabetes have a raised incidence of depression, especially around the time of diagnosis. The new GP contract acknowledges the increased prevalence of the disease and requires GPs to screen this patient group annually. There are many instruments that are suitable for screening patients for depression. The most commonly used questionnaire in general practice is the PHQ-9 (see Table in Case 62). Emotional disturbances, depression and a stressful home or work environment are common reasons why patients do not respond to treatment.

 KEY POINTS

- The health professional–patient relationship can become a burden for health professionals, especially when they try hard to help patients. It is important to notice when a patient becomes a 'heart-sink patient' and ask for help from colleagues.
- Emotional problems in patients are a common cause for failure to respond to treatment.

History

The GP is consulted by a 15-year-old girl who presents with her mother. Her mother has made her come along because she has noticed a marked weight loss in her daughter over the past few weeks. She has also noticed that her daughter seems pale and unwell. Normally, when she presents to the surgery the young woman wears baggy clothes and is not forthcoming, and there have been times when the GP has suspected an eating disorder. The patient's body mass index (BMI) hovers around 19, but an eating disorder has always been denied by the patient and her mother. The GP has never noticed the patient being as thin as she is now. The patient has a younger brother of 12 years of age and they live with their parents in the local estate. The girl has not had any serious illness but the GP has seen her on a number of occasions with minor disorders such as sore throats and coughs and colds. It appears that she and her mother do not get along very well but it has never been possible to work out what is really going on. It has been frustrating and worrying for the GP who has taken the situation to the surgery clinical meetings on a number of occasions but the practice has not been able to get to the bottom of the problem.

The GP assumes that the girl is suffering from a worsening of the suspected eating disorder and hopes that this time they will finally be able to tackle the problem. However, on questioning the girl further the GP is surprised when the girl tells her that she has been feeling really thirsty recently and passing lots of urine, even getting up at night a few times to go to the toilet.

Questions
• What is the probable diagnosis?
• What does the GP do now?
• What should the GP be concerned about in the months that follow?

ANSWER

With the classic signs of polydypsia, polyuria and weight loss the girl probably has Type 1 diabetes mellitus.

The GP finds glucose and ketones in the urine and a finger-prick blood glucose reports 'HI'. The girl's BMI is now down to 17. With signs of ketoacidosis the GP refers her straight to hospital where it is found that she has borderline acidosis and ketosis, a blood sugar of 34 mmol/L and an HbA1C (glycated haemoglobin) of 15.8 per cent. The patient is admitted from casualty for treatment and she started on insulin: human Insulatard twice a day and insulin aspart three times a day before meals. She is also fully informed by the diabetic nurse specialist and the dietitian about her condition and its management. After 14 days her blood glucose control has improved dramatically and the patient is changed from insulin aspart to NovoRapid and remains on a reduced dose of Insulatard twice a day. Diabetic retinal screening and foot examination are normal. The diabetic clinic plans to refer her to the 5-day DAFNE programme (Dose Adjustment for Normal Eating) at 6 months, after the initial period of attempting best control.

The GP must still keep in mind the possibility of an eating disorder as well as the diabetes. An eating disorder and Type 1 diabetes in a teenage girl is a dangerous mix. It has been estimated that one in three young women with diabetes abuse their insulin, missing injections to stay thin, leading to a greatly increased risk of diabetic complications. This young patient needs rapid access to psychological care and support, with close monitoring to help her manage her condition effectively. The GP hopes that the diabetes has at least given a way in to treating other family and psychological problems.

 KEY POINTS

- Keep your mind open to possibilities when eliciting a history.
- Signs of ketoacidosis in a patient with suspected diabetes mellitus require urgent referral to hospital.
- 'Diabulimia' as it has been termed – missing injections to stay thin – is a common and dangerous condition in young women with diabetes.

INDEX

References are by case number with relevant page number(s) following in brackets. References with a page range e.g. 25(68-70) indicate that although the subject may be mentioned only on one page, it concerns the whole case. Page numbers for Figures are indicated in italics; that in bold type indicates a Table.